THE

TELEVISION

Edward Lee

A Madness Heart Press Publication

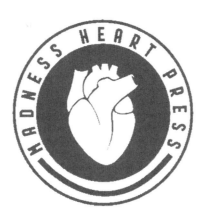

Madness Heart Press
2006 Idlewilde Run Dr.
Austin, Texas 78744

This is a work of fiction. Names, characters, places, and incidents either are the product of the author's imagination or are used fictitiously. Any resemblance to actual persons, living or dead, events, or locales is entirely coincidental.

Copyright © 2022 Edward Lee
Cover by John Baltisberger

All rights reserved. No part of this book may be reproduced or used in any manner without written permission of the copyright owner except for the use of quotations in a book review. For more information, address: john@madnessheart. press

First Edition
ISBN: 978-1-955745-28-4
www.madnessheart.press

Acknowledgements

John Baltisberger, Christine Morgan, Lisa Tone, Jackie, Gina, Matt Shaw, Roman and Artur, John Newton, Jaime, Nickolay Cusev, Brad Tierney, Patrick and Brennan at Dead Headspace, Craig Steele, Mark Goddard, Demonika, Erik Smith, Phobophile, Blurb, Plagued by Visions, Plaguelands Media, Emily Drzal Lasater

THE TELEVISION

The old man in the chair sat in tinted, buzzy darkness, as he'd sat many, many times before, enthralled by what wonders the screen would reveal: those delicious visions, those ever-potent images that circumvented age and infirmity.

How many times had he done this?

His slugging heart told him this would be the last.

So make it a good one, old chap!

He'd already emptied the goblet, immune to the nausea it compelled. His pants were open; his ancient cock was out and erect as an eighteen-year-old's. His crabbed hand wrapped around it and squeezed; he could feel the pulse beating. *How about just one more for old time's sake, eh? For posterity?* If anything, his cock got harder at the thought, and he smiled. *One more for the His Majesty the King?*

His mouth went dry as he stared at the screen, which depicted a large, antiquated bulldozer plowing through a twenty-foot-high pile of emaciated, naked corpses. Male and female alike, the heads of the corpses had all been shaved, and they lolled there as if disjointed; they were skin-covered skeletons, sunken-eyed, slat-ribbed. The dozer's operator sat tiny up at the controls, aghast, a rag tied over his mouth and nose. He backed the machine up to plow another swath of the human mountain.

Aside, two soldiers with gas masks waded into the pile; they were hunting for the freshest female corpses, and eventually, they pulled two out— adolescent girls, by the looks of them, their mouths frozen open in eternal screams.

The two soldiers dropped their trousers and began to rape the pair of corpses.

It was at this point that the old man in the chair began to frenetically masturbate.

"Ah, yes," said a hefty British voice on the phone. "I'm in dire need of contacting one Mr. I. W. Farthing, son of Wilma and John Farthing."

Farthing was distracted. The brunt of his

attention was now devoted to his computer screen; he was at this moment engaged in watching an old Barbara Steele movie, *Terror Creatures From The Grave*. There was a bathtub scene in which Ms. Steele, covered in suds, betrayed, for one infinitesimal split-second, a bare nipple. Trust any Barbara Steele fan: it was a moment worth waiting for, and that's exactly what Farthing was doing when his budget-brand flip-style cellphone rang. *Fuck! he thought of the interruption.* "Yes, I'm I. W. Farthing," *he snapped.*

"Born in Wheaton, Maryland, on February first, nineteen—?"

"Yes, don't remind me ..." Farthing rolled his eyes. Barbara's nipple had come and gone. He'd have to rewind. "Who is this?"

"My name is Montague Cooper, and I am the solicitor for—"

"Solicitor?" Farthing couldn't get away from them! "I'm on the Do Not Call List, damn it! Don't you people even *look* at that anymore? It's a terrible business model to call people when you *know* they don't want to be called! Get a regular job instead of one that pesters people to buy things they don't want! Whatever it is you're selling, I *don't want it.* If I did, I'd go to the *store* and buy it. I don't need some snide charlie ringing my phone to try to sell it to me. Fuck, last week one of you guys called to ask if I wanted my basement waterproofed, and I don't even *have* a fuckin' basement! I *hate* phone solicitors!"

A long pause seemed to indicate befuddlement after Farthing's tirade. "I'm afraid there's a misunderstanding, Mr. Farthing. I most decidedly am *not* a telephone solicitor. I'm calling from England, and I'm no less than the attorney for your uncle on your father's side—"

Farthing's brow shot up. "Uncle Eldred?"

"Yes, sir, and since it's unlikely you've already been otherwise notified, I'm afraid I have the regrettable duty to alert you to the fact that a little less than two months or so ago, your Uncle Eldred met upon his decease."

Farthing made a face. "You mean he died?"

"Yes, sir. At his home in eastern England, sir, in the town of Burnstow."

This left Farthing immediately depressed, in spite of having never once met Uncle Eldred. "What sucky news," he muttered. "He and I have exchanged birthday and Christmas cards for …" *Damn, I'm getting old* … "I'll bet over fifty years. And we did speak on the phone once or twice back when my mother was still alive. He seemed like a nice guy …" Farthing's lips pursed. *And now he's a nice DEAD guy.* Farthing was in his sixties now, so he could only guess that Uncle Eldred was in his nineties when his "golden bowl" had "ceased to vibrate."

"A man of eccentrical habits, perhaps," Cooper remarked, "but indeed a very *nice guy,* as you would say, and obviously a man with some considerable feelings of kindliness toward you, Mr. Farthing. His will names you as his sole heir …"

Farthing's eyes shot wide as he instantly envisioned a sprawling Victorian manse sitting atop a grand hill and overlooking a hundred or so acres of plush pastures and venerable trees—that and a long garage full of Rolls Royces.

Cooper continued, "And mightn't I add that Eldred was a man of some financial means? I knew him personally and can say that I was not only his attorney but also a personal friend. A generous man was he, always willing to give to the community charities or slip a ten to a homeless type. But you'll remember when, a moment ago, I referred to him as a man with an eccentrical bent? While possessed of an impressive financial endowment, he chose to live in a mobile home, in a static mobile home park."

Farthing's mouth fell open and, indeed, so did Barbara Steele's at the precise moment of that unseemly revelation. There went the Victorian manse and the Rolls Royces. Farthing lived in a mobile home himself, one that was built in 1967. Men of "impressive financial endowments" did *not live in trailers. Fuck,* he thought.

"Hence my reference to eccentricities." Cooper chuckled. "The mobile home is all yours now, along with everything in it, including some rare bits of furniture, some antiques, and a shelf or two of very old and very valuable books, barely anything—he told me once—later than the mid-1800s—"

Farthing frowned. On his monitor, Barbara Steele was out of the tub and quickly wrapping herself in a robe while arguing with a cute blonde.

"—not to mention a stipend of 3000 pounds per month for as long as you shall live."

Farthing nearly fell off his seat, his heart slamming. "Whuh-what—How much is 3000 pounds in duh-duh-dollars?"

"Today? About $3700," Mr. Cooper informed.

"Per month, you said?"

"Per month, Mr. Farthing. For the rest of your life."

Barbara Steele was forgotten. Farthing's brain ticked. *God bless Uncle Eldred!* That money along with his Social Security would exponentially improve the quality of his life. "This almost sounds … too good to be true …"

"Oh, it's true," Cooper assured him. "And if you'd be so good as to give me your email, I'll send you all the pertinent data."

This Farthing did, his mind still jumbled by the shock of what he'd just been told. *I won't have to live like a pauper anymore! I can get Uber Eats and everything! And I can move out of this fuckin' piece of shit trailer!*

"But there is one legal stipulation related to what your uncle has bestowed upon you, the unwaiverable provision that you relocate here to East Suffolk and *live* in your uncle's mobile home — that is, if you want to collect your stipend."

Farthing felt like a floor safe had just been dropped on his head. "You mean I get nothing unless I move to fuckin' *England?*"

An unappreciative pause. "That's quite correct, sir, and you must *take up residence in your uncle's trailer.*"

"Can't I just sell it!" Farthing blurted.

"Oh, but of course," Cooper clarified. "And my firm would be more than happy to help you with that. But if you do, you inherit nothing else. And I'm afraid the trailer — the mobile home — isn't worth very much of itself. I mean, how *can* it be?"

Cooper chuckled again. "It's a mobile home."

Farthing frowned, looking around at the shambles of his own trailer. *Great ...* "But if I *did sell* my uncle's trailer, who gets the three thousand a month?"

"I'm afraid in *that* case, the entirety of your uncle's liquid assets would be donated, in a lump sum, to the Ontology Department of Cambridge University," Cooper replied. "However, before making so weighty a decision, Mr. Farthing, why not step round for a visit? Make an assessment of your potential property. Introduce yourself to the neighborhood, and at least spend a few nights in your belated uncle's abode. Of course, we will pay for your trip. Hmm?"

Farthing let out a long breath, casting another glance at Barbara Steele's whopping cleavage, and then he rendered his answer to Cooper ...

It would unfairly task the reader's patience to elaborate on the precise sequence of events that led to the deposition of Farthing's butt upon a stool at the Mattshaw Pub in the sedate oceanfront town of Burnstow, England. *What's a Mattshaw? he wondered. Is it like a rickshaw?* At any rate, said deposition occurred not even a fortnight from the

11

time he'd received his phone call from Mr. Cooper, informing him of his uncle's demise, etc., etc. Cooper's suggestion that he—Farthing—acquaint himself with the town and the mobile home before making any further decisions really seemed like the best idea.

And now we find him in the pre-assigned pub, waiting for Mr. Cooper.

Farthing supposed the pub was just like *any* English pub he'd seen in the movies: lots of dark wood and brass, heavy tables and chairs, and something of a nautical motif. A long row of beer taps followed down the bartop.

A stout though shapely woman—fiftyish perhaps—proffering a consequential bosom and a name tag that read Bernice, approached him with a stolid smile. "What'll it be?"

Farthing's eyes surveyed the long row of beer taps; nothing familiar looked back at him. "No Budweiser, I see. What's the closest thing you've got to Budweiser?"

The barmaid huffed a laugh. "Now don't you take offense by what I say to ya, sir. But the closest thing we got to Budweiser? Here? Is the door."

I guess that's British hospitality ... "Whatever you've got that's cheap."

"Ah, that's just what we like round here, sir,"

Bernice said huskily. "A big spender! Comin' right up."

No one else occupied the bar, which Farthing attributed to the early hour. *Only drunks drink at noon,* he thought, then sipped the beer that had been placed before him.

"My word," said Bernice, giving him the eye. "And what might your name be? Farthing, is it?"

"Well, yes," Farthing replied. "How did you know?"

"You must be Eldred Farthing's kin. You look just like 'im. He never once mentioned a son."

"He doesn't have one. He's my uncle—er, was."

"Yes, I 'eard he passed, but as old as he was?"

"Yeah. If I make it to seventy, I'll be happy." The beer was strong but smooth. "And as for any resemblance, this is the first I've heard of it. You see, I never met my uncle and I don't remember ever seeing a picture of him."

"Well, you're the spittin' image, I can tell ya."

"Anyway, I'm here to see the place where he lived."

"The mobile home, aye. 'Tis a nice park," Bernice offered, or perhaps she was just trying to sound positive.

"So I take it you knew my uncle fairly well?" Farthing ventured.

"Well enough—" Did she grin? "—back in the day, I should say."

He didn't know how to assess the remark, but his dirty mind made plenty of suggestions. *Ten, twenty years ago? I'll bet she was something. And with THOSE tits?* But such instant ruminations were a social debilitation from being single his entire adult life. He couldn't help it.

"Plannin' on stayin'?" she asked, washing pint glasses.

"I—I …"

"Or just havin' a look about, I imagine."

Farthing was "havin' a look" at Bernice's bosom, each breast big as a baby's head. *Can you IMAGINE the nipples?* he asked himself. "Yes, this is more of a scouting expedition," he compared. "I'll figure it out as I go. Maybe I'll move here, maybe I won't. Can you tell me what I might expect when I get to my uncle's trailer?"

Bernice shrugged. "A mobile home's a mobile home, ya ask me. Eldred were nice as the day is long, I can say, but—"

Farthing looked up. "Eccentric?"

"Yeah. What I mean is it's everyone's question 'ow a man that rich live in a mobile home, and why ain't no one never seen him drivin' a car? Lord knows he could afford one."

"Well … Are you certain he was rich?"

"Now, sir, I ain't sayin' we'se all a bunch of snoops here," Bernice asserted, standing up straight. This change in position only elucidated Farthing's view of her bosom. "And a town like this—small's, what I mean. Close-knit. Little bits of things 'ave their way of being whispered here 'n' whispered there, and like, someone maybe workin' in the bank might accidentally see his balance, and someone workin' a table at the Lamplighter might catch a glimpse of one 'a them black American Express cards, and someone else might 'a seen him at the harness track bettin' enough cash money ta sink the Queen Mary. Like that."

Farthing nodded. *Snoops. Just like Americans …*

Now Bernice sat on her own stool behind the bar, leaning forward slightly. This position only served to *further* elucidate her giant breasts, leaving Farthing to imagine them bare. *June Palmer? he thought. No. Bigger. Dyanne Thorne? Yeah. But not quite a Chesty Morgan …* Farthing considered that she might be effecting that pose on purpose, not because she was attracted to him but … *She might have an interest in a naive newcomer about to inherit some money. But what a thing to think!*

"And then there were his cronies," Bernice continued, "and I can tell you, *that* made talk."

"Cronies?"

"Oh, yeah, some high-rollers, these blokes were." Bernice seemed amused. "Eldred said they was all part of some sorta travel club, but that didn't really mesh. All the time I knowed that man, I can't remember once he ever set foot outta this town, and I known 'im must be forty years."

This sounded interesting. "High-rollers, you say? Some sort of a club?"

Bernice nodded; she poured herself the tiniest sip of some liquor, shot it back, then the glass was gone like a magic trick. "Least that what he say. Forig men, a lot of them was, all with the accents and some with right funny clothes."

Farthing listened with attentiveness, getting that *forig must mean foreign.*

She went on. "One tall fella as black as coal, I 'eard he was some sorta diplomat from Sennergull or some such, some African place, and some Norway fella who owned oil wells 'n' come in a yacht, and then another fella, a Russian, and next day Doris the food runner show me a magazine with the bloke's picture in it, and it turn out he was one 'a them hoolah-garks, Vitaly something, his name was, and there was his pitcher right there in the magazine, a *billionaire,* it say." Bernice cut out a high laugh. "Can you reckon it? A bloody *billionaire comin' here?"*

"And others?" Farthing asked. "Other rich guys, all friends with my uncle?"

"That's a fact. It were everyone's question for years: what's such an odd mix 'a well-to-do gents coming here from God knows where, just ta visit Eldred, a old Brit, drink with him in this bloody pub, and then go back ta his *trailer,* for bloody sake? A pretty rum thing, ya ask me."

Well, maybe it *wasn't a "rum" thing, really. Uncle Eldred merely had a diverse congregation of friends ...* and Farthing doubted very seriously that any *billionaires were in the bunch. People had a way*—especially *village* folk—of fabricating. Nevertheless, it piqued Farthing's interest and would be something to make inquiry to Cooper about, whenever he got here—

A cowbell jangled; Farthing could feel light on his back when the pub door opened.

"Ah, there he is," Bernice announced a bit loudly. "Here is your gentleman, Mr. Cooper, what I think you know. I just been givin' him a proper greeting to our 'umble little town."

Farthing stood up and turned to see a short, rotund man—dark-haired, balding, and with a round trimmed beard—hurry forward with an extended hand.

"Mr. Farthing, such a pleasure to meet you, and I'm glad Bernice has properly greeted you; of course, I only wish I could've been the first to render a greeting myself were it not for a low front tire." Cooper shook Farthing's hand heartily. The man, in his neat, dark suit and tie, reminded Farthing of Sebastian Cabot (Farthing was old enough to know who that was.). "You'll forgive me for staring, sir, but the resemblance betwixt yourself and your uncle is extraordinary."

"Yes, Bernice just pointed that out. Hi, how are you—"

"And may your arrival here," Cooper cheerily continued, "be marked as a red letter day! Bernice, be so kind as to put Mr. Farthing's libation on my account." He picked up Farthing's suitcase. "And now, sir, if you're ready, let us go investigate your uncle's abode, shall we?"

Farthing downed his beer and nodded at the same time, then followed Cooper to the door.

"I do hope you'll come again!" Bernice called after them.

Farthing glanced back and waved. *What great tits ...*

But a bit distant from the Mattshaw Pub, something very different was afoot. It need not be diagnosticated exactly where the following introduction was taking place. Let's just imagine that if you divided a map of England into four quarters, the area in question would be located in the southwestern quadrant. And it was here, in a place of employment, that an attractive thirtyish woman with small, hard breasts, multicolored hair, and spectacular tan lines, named Mal—short for Malison—was working her next customer in what the business parlance referred to as a "shop." No, it was not a candy shop, a coffee shop, or anything of *that* kind. It was, instead— at least according to the license on the wall—an "aromatherapy" shop, where clients would come to "relax" while an attractive, barely clothed woman—with an "aromatherapy" license, mind you—would light fragrant candles and apply various "aromatherapy" essential oils—lavender, eucalyptus, orange extracts, etc.—to the patron's body. The combination of pleasant scents along with the relaxing environment would supposedly improve sleep, relieve headaches and other types of pain, eliminate stress, and boost energy.

And if you believe *that* bullshit, I know an author who's got a bridge to sell you. Next time you're driving around and you see a little shop with a sign that reads AROMATHERAPY, if you think it's really a place for aromatherapy, you're nothing less than an idiot. It's a fuckin' *whorehouse.*

This particular whorehouse was called FULL MOON, and Mal had worked there for several years, since she'd been dishonorably separated from the Royal Air Force for gang-banging—for money, of course—a platoon of SA 300 helicopter mechanics. So much for *that* career, and she hadn't even had an orgasm, which seemed howlingly unfair.

Mal specialized in any aspect of whoredom, but specifically "dominatrix" services. There was a certain class of men who paid *untold* sums of money to be humiliated, insulted, mocked, restrained, and, in one way or other, have their asses *kicked* by domineering women. Such desires, say the experts, hearkened back to childhood anomalies, or perhaps that's just a modern-day manner of beating around the bush. Maybe they were simply *born* fucked up in the head.

At this precise moment, Mal was "breaking in" a new employee, a pert nineteen-year-old with long jet-black hair, named Darcy. Both Darcy and Mal stood unabashedly naked in front of the pathetic, also naked customer, a palish, shortish, stoutish man going bald. He sort of just hung there before the two women because he'd been, per his own request, lashed by the ankles and wrists to a sturdy wooden X, taller than him. His shrinking genitals barely showed themselves beneath the sagging pallid belly.

"Get a load of this switch-hitter, will ya, love?" Mal said to Darcy, though eyeing the very despondent-looking client before them. "This bloke paid seven-fifty for the works. Number Six on the menu, can ya believe it?"

Darcy's pretty face lengthened in astonishment. *"Damn, that's a lot of money. But …* what's Number Six?"

"Learn the menu, hon. It's part 'a your responserbility, it is." Breaking new girls in at a place like Full Moon was always some extra effort. "You ever done Dom?"

"Huh?"

Jeeze. "In a place like this, these chubnuts want to be *dominated* by women. They want to be insulted, spat on, roughed up. Get it?"

"Uh, yeah, I think."

Mal frowned. "Where'd you work before this?"

"Silver Key—"

"Honey, that's just a jack-shack. I worked there when I was sixteen, bet I wanked a couple

21

thousand blokes there. That shit's small-time. So you've never done Dom or S&M?"

"Uh, well—"

"Where you used ta work, babe, is the farm league compared to Full Moon. These ain't no fifty-quid handjobs. Here, it's the real sickos that lay down righteous cash to get what they want, 'cos they sure as a brown trout ain't gettin' it at home." Mal nodded with self-assurance, still eyeing the client. "Most of 'em? They'se millionaires, they are. They're CEO's and all that, they run big companies 'n' order people around all day. Perfect little shits, like this fatso here. Probably fires people for fun— just 'cos he *can*—fires folks with kids ta raise, makes 'em feel like big men." She pinched the client's cheeks and made fish-lips on his face. "But then they come 'ere because deep-down there ain't nothin' they want more 'n' ta be punished by their mommies or daddies, ain't that right, arsehole?" Mal slapped the web of her hand against his throat and squeezed so hard the client began to squirm. "Answer me when I talk to you, fruit-face, or you can bet your favorite butt-plug I will *fuck you up*."

The client gasped, "Yes, yes, you're right, miss—"

"Well, you are one chubbly-wubbly, ain't ya? And would ya *look* at these man-tits? Shit, buddy, you got tits on ya bigger 'n' most women." She *slapped her open hands on his chest and began to knead the fat there. "Yeah, I'll bet ya like* that, don't ya, you fat fairy-boy, you *like* me feelin' up these big hairy tits on ya. Well, just let's see how ya like *this ..." and then* Mal's mouth opened, her face shot forward, and she clamped her front teeth down hard on one of his nipples.

The client tensed up on the X and nearly howled from the pain.

Mal looked down at the man's crotch with a half-grin and a half-grimace. "See what I mean, hon?" she asked Darcy. "That's how fucked up in the head these blokes are. I practically bit his bloomin' nipple off, and he pulls a hard-on!"

Darcy couldn't believe her eyes. After all that pain and humiliation, the man's cock had sprung fully erect and was pulsing.

"But that's just the appetizer," Mal explained, "not the main course. We like to fuck with 'em a bit first, just ta get 'em going, ya know?" Before she could say more, there came a repeated muffled sound from the next room, like—

fwump! fwump! fwump!

—but in between each *fwump,* there was a loud disorganized groan occurring in tandem with a hacking, gagging sound.

fwump! fwump! fwump!

Darcy shot Mal a fretful glance. "What—what's that?"

"Oh, that ain't but Harriet workin' over a customer. See, she's our resident ball-buster."

Darcy's eyes widened. "Buh-ball—"

"Harriet was in college on a sports scholarship; she was on the women's soccer team," Mal explained, "but, well, you know how it goes. She got expelled on account she was selling pills on campus. So she come ta us for a job and fit right in. See, hon, there are fellas out there who'll pay for anything, and one 'a them things is, they'll pay a girl to kick 'em in the balls. Now, I don't mean like pretend kicks or little baby kicks. I mean they pay for the girl to kick 'em in the bollocks *hard, over and over—*"

fwump! fwump! fwump!

"—and I mean so hard these blokes are curled up on the floor cryin' and suckin' their thumbs."

"But, but—It must hurt like all hell!"

"Sure it does, love. That's what they'se paying for. For the pain. They're bloody masochists. Only way these numpties can even cum is if they're doubled-over in agony. That's how fucked up they are." Mal chuckled. "Last year I 'member Harriet had this pillock of a customer who was in the foreign service, he was, and he come in here and pay her to kick his balls like there's no tomorrow. And she kept kickin' and kickin', and he keep say 'harder, harder!' and she say she kicked his balls so many times her fuckin' *foot* started to hurt, so she lay back and give him one more kick and— POW! You know what happened?"

Darcy's mouth fell open. "He ... he died?"

fwump! fwump! fwump!

Mal frowned. "No, for fuck's sake, he didn't *die,* but she sure as fuck ruptured the motherfucker. His nut, like, *popped,* it did, and it come kind of *unwound* like a golf ball do when the cover's cut, and this silly shit-head's standin' there howling at the moon with his ball-sack all swollen up the size of a bag of fuckin' marshmallows!"

"Holy shit!" Darcy exclaimed. "Did he have to get surgery?"

"No, no, hon. He just left it, and in a month or so, it all come back together and healed." Mal nodded, arms crossed. "And it wasn't too long after that, the same twisted bloke come right back in here and pay Harriet to bust his other one."

"No!"

"I ain't makin' this shit up, love. Men are so much more fucked up than women, you can't even believe it." Mal cast another glance at the client,

25

and it would be fair to refer to the look on her face as an expression sheer unfiltered disgust. "And now we got this sissy-pants turd-burglar wantin' a Number Six from the menu." She pinched his cheeks again. "Well, we here at Full Moon, we aim ta please, and you're gonna get *exactly* what ya paid for, you sick, twisted, pathetic, fat *bastard.*" And then she shot forward and bit him again hard on his nipple.

He bellowed high and hard.

Mal went to a metal cabinet and opened some drawers.

Darcy gulped, and finally, the burning question was asked again. "What's ... Number Six?"

"A double-cath," Mal replied, "not that I suspect you know what that is. Know what a catheter is?"

Darcy stared, her mouth still hanging open. "Uh, something—oh, you mean like a heart catheter? My gramps had one!"

Mal's smirk told all. "No, love. Not a heart catheter." She held up several plastic bags from the drawer. One's front read URINARY CATHETER (PRE-LUBRICATED). She threw Darcy the other bag.

Darcy looked shocked. This bag read ENEMA KIT. "Aw, no ..."

"Yep," Mal said cheerily. "But the way we do it

here? 'Tis different. Now, open that bag and pull out the tube."

Trepidatiously, she withdrew the rolled-up tube complete with the enema nozzle on the end. The actual enema bag remained unconnected to the tube.

"We ain't gonna be needin' the water bag, hon, just the tube an nozzle," Mal instructed. She pointed to a one-pound jar of Vaseline on the cabinet. "Now lube up the nozzle with some Vaseline, and don't be skimpy."

Darcy did as instructed with a long look on her face. Her hands were shaking.

"Come on, love. If you wanna do this job, you gotta do it with confidence. Act like ya know your way about. And when you're done, stick that nozzle in this loser's arsehole."

"Oh-oh my …" Darcy muttered, her hands shaking. She falteringly pushed open one of the client's butt cheeks … "It's just so, so *gross.*"

"Ain't much more in this here whole world grosser than a bloke's hairy arsecrack, love. Makes ya just wanna kill 'em, don't it? But if you want the money, just you stick that nozzle in there right now."

After several starts, Darcy managed the task. The client flinched and then moaned with pleasure as the nozzle sank in. The process left him with a tube hanging out of his ass like a tail.

"So-so what do we do now?" Darcy asked. "Fill the rubber bag with water and squirt it up his ass?"

Mal flapped a hand. "No, no, dear. Ya really must leave it to me. Watch and learn." She grinned at Darcy. "First thing we gotta do is empty the fat bastard's bladder. And if you're a perceptive type, Doris—"

"Darcy," Darcy corrected.

"Right. Sorry. But like I was sayin', if you're the perceptive type, you should be looking 'round and thinkin' to yourself, 'Where the bloody hell is this chump gonna empty his bladder? I don't see no toilet in this room.' Is that somethin' like what you're thinkin'?"

Darcy was beside herself. "Well, yeah …"

Mal raised a finger. "And *that's* where you're wrong, hon, because, ya see, there very much *is* a toilet in this room," and then she pointed her finger directly at the client.

Darcy didn't get it. "What—"

"*He's* the fuckin' toilet, love. In fact, the way I see it, *all men are toilets! Now watch 'cos you're gonna have to do this on your own soon.*"

First Mal took the back end of the catheter and connected it to the end of the enema tube going into the client's ass. Then she took the plastic cover off the pre-lubricated urinary catheter, then positioned herself with authority before the shuddering client. With the thumb and forefinger of one hand, she lifted up the end of the man's penis, and with the thumb and forefinger of her other hand, she tweezed the end of the catheter, and—

"No!" Darcy exclaimed, her fists to her chin.

Mal slowly slid the catheter up into the client's penis, the sensation of which urged the client to flex his hips and moan as if in deep pleasure.

"When ya get to the end," Mal continued, "ya gotta *push,* you know, kind of *nudge it through so's it go straight into the bloke's bladder, and there! See!" The catheter instantly filled with urine. She fish-lipped the client again, pinching hard. "Now piss*, you silly-arse tubesteak! Piss *hard!"*

The client was pissing, all right, exerting those urinary muscles and sending his piss from his bladder right up his ass. He continued to moan through the process. Eventually, no more urine could be seen filling the catheter.

"Good boy, you sick fat plonker!" Mal celebrated. "And now for the best part. Diana, er, Darcy—that's the name, ain't it? Just you come over here right now and pinch off that enema tube, and then separate the tube from the catheter. Pinch hard now 'cos we can't have all the piss up this schmuck's arse emptyin' on the floor, now can we?"

Darcy was incapable of response and was beginning to think that maybe the Full Moon wasn't the right place for her to seek employment, money or not. Nevertheless, she pinched off the enema tube and disconnected it from the original catheter.

"There ya go," Mal complimented. "You're gettin' the hang 'a this right quick, you are! Now pull that filthy thing out of this bastard's butt and throw it out."

When Darcy did this, gritting her teeth in disgust, the client flinched again and groaned.

This left the original catheter sticking out of the client's penis, a sight of supreme hilarity. Next, Mal opened a second catheter and connected its rearend to the end of the catheter sticking out of the client's dick. Astute readers will not need further exposition; but for the less astute ... here we go.

Mal stood, feet apart, opened *another* catheter and connected its backend to the catheter sticking out of the client's dick. Then she V'd open her vulva where she stood. Her fingers fiddled around inside, she said, "Ah, there it is," and stuck the lubricated end of the *new* catheter into the opening of her own urethra. She slid the clear plastic tube deep, deep, deeper until — "There we are!" — she'd successfully catheterized her own bladder (which, it might be added, was quite full from the two pints of beer she'd had for lunch). Instantly, of course, this new catheter filled with Mal's urine, and then her stomach muscles tensed as she pushed her own piss into the client's bladder with racehorse force. Even Darcy watched amazed as the area between the client's belly button and cock began to distend.

Mal extended a hand to the pathetic, shivering excuse of a client. "Now *that* is what we call the Number Six on the menu, love," and then she addressed the client directly and fish-lipped him yet again. "All happy now, you ridiculous pervert? Now ya got your backside all filled up with your own piss and your bladder all filled up with mine! Bet you'll slosh like a barrel of ale when you waddle out of here."

Darcy staggered behind Mal to the breakroom; she looked shell-shocked.

Mal nodded. "See? Nothin' to it. The money's worth the inconvenience, and the guy coming in next is payin' even more than that fat bald pussy."

Darcy only half-heard her. "You mean …

another Number Six?"

"No, hon, it's a Number Four, and double fisting. But don't worry, we get to wear rubber gloves."

Darcy gulped, made a kind of chirp in the back of her throat, and made a quick exit from the building.

Mal shrugged, and to herself said, "Kids these days. They're all a bunch of sissies and mollycoddles …"

It was not a Rolls Royce that awaited them outside but a Bentley. Cooper, clearly, was a successful lawyer.

"You'll see on our way," Cooper enlightened, "that our nice little seaside town is equipped with pretty much all you might need. A grocer's, a pharmacy, several eateries—oh, and in our little bank"—Cooper pointed to the squat brick building that read BURNSTOW TRUST—"I've opened you an account where your monthly payment will be direct-deposited in the event you decide to remain with us. Two months have accrued already."

"That sounds … marvelous," Farthing said, a little shocked. *My British account already has more than my US account, and I haven't been here an hour*

...

"I believe everything you're likely to need awaits you—everything, that is, except company."

Farthing looked over at Cooper behind the wheel; he was already weirded out by the car being on the wrong side of the road. "I'm not much of a people person, Mr. Cooper. All I need is my cable TV."

"Well, that we have, sir, Netflix, Amazon, various subscription services. It's all set up and so is the Wi-Fi."

"I feel at home already," Farthing said with a smile. But as they drove down the little town's Main Street, he noticed that their passing turned a good many pedestrian heads. This told him that stock was being taken of him, which lent him a turn of paranoia. *Hey, everyone. Here comes the new guy—an American ...*

As they drove along, Cooper smiled and tipped an imaginary hat to the present town folk.

"Mr. Cooper? Bernice said something curious, something about my Uncle Eldred being in some sort of club? A travel club, maybe? She said my uncle had a lot of rich friends, billionaires, even."

Cooper chuckled. "It is true, Mr. Farthing, that your late uncle did indeed belong to a club—not a *travel* club, to my knowledge—but an alumni club.

Eldred was a Cambridge man quite some time ago. Did you know he was nearly a hundred when he passed? I think you can be assured of good genes! And, yes, he had many such friends who also attended Cambridge, but of course, they're all much younger. And are they rich? Well, yes, a good many of them are—after all, they graduated from Cambridge—quite like your Harvard—and some of them became, you could say, Captains of Industry. But ... billionaires?" Another chuckle. "Not likely. Just a bunch of drinking buddies really. They'd get together three, four times a year, like that is all. Bernice—I've not a single word to say against her—might have a leaning toward hyperbole, if you know what I mean."

Tall tales, Farthing thought. He knew that by living so many years at his own trailer park: when people got bored, they made up stories, or they saw things that weren't really there. He hoped *he* never became like that.

"And there's my office, sir." Cooper pointed to another squat brick building; a sign read COOPER'S ATTORNEYS AT LAW. "I'm proud to say that I'm the senior partner"—another of his ubiquitous chuckles—"as well as the *only partner. I'd be happy to avail myself to all your legal needs. If you want to sue someone"*—he raised a finger—"I'm your man, sir.

Dastardly, aren't we? Like Shakespeare said, *Kill all the lawyers,* eh? A word or two of wisdom for us all, Shakespeare—that's what my poor father used to say. 'There are more things in Heaven and earth …'"

Farthing, born into a blue-collar world, had worked thirty-five years at a cardboard box factory. He didn't know from Shakespeare. The only Hamlet he knew was the Hamburger Hamlet in Tampa. "Would you happen to know if this park has a rat problem?" he asked. "Every so often, mine back in Florida becomes infested."

"'Tis a funny place for rats is your uncle's court," Cooper explained. "I've never heard of so much as a single rodent showing its furry face, which you might expect since so many residents own cats. Oh, and that reminds me—the Cat Lady. There are a few noteworthy residents at the park—"

"The Cat Lady?" Farthing asked. He could only imagine.

"Yes. I've not a word to say against her, nor have I any clue as to her name. I only know she lives somewhere on your uncle's street, and every evening at various times, she emerges from her mobile home and walks up and down the road talking on her cellphone. She has at least a half-dozen cats following her, and when she's done with her calls, she talks to them—the cats, that is."

Farthing shrugged. At his own trailer park, there was far worse than the Cat Lady. There was the couple across the street, nearing their eighties, who bellowed at each other at all hours, raving profanities the likes of which might make Caligula raise a brow. Then there was the oldster next door who walked his ancient dog at night, a dog which howled at the moon whenever it defecated—often in Farthing's lot—because of doggie hemorrhoids. Not to mention another elderly man who thought nothing of putting out his garbage in only jockey shorts. Yes, trailer life was something. "I think I can hack the Cat Lady."

Cooper winked. "Late-forties or so, and not hard on the eyes, if you receive my meaning."

This perked Farthing up. Positive human imagery was more than welcome—especially since there was so little of it at a retirement park. *Night of the Living Old People,* he thought, but he supposed he was one of the old people himself, one of the zombies.

"And until recently, there was the Piss Car Lady—"

"The *what?*" Farthing gawped at Cooper.

"Drat, I suppose I shouldn't have mentioned it. She hasn't been seen in months, died, they say, of old age, which is a blessing if you'd ever seen her."

"Yeah, but … the *Piss Car* Lady?" With a name like that … Farthing just *had* to know.

"Well, your uncle knew her most of her life; she grew up here in town, and from a family of good circumstances. But you know how it goes for some. Hard times fell upon her; your uncle even implied she was, as they say, a lady of the night, for as long as her looks would manage it. Eventually, she became homeless. Her fifties came and went, her sixties, like that. She was living in her car, and they called her the Piss Car Lady because, well, whenever she'd drive by anyone, you could smell it. It must've been dirty laundry she kept piled up in the backseat, or maybe she became incontinent and—you know—just said to Hades with it and soiled herself where she sat. I'm afraid she'd come by the trailer park looking for handouts, the poor girl, and your uncle was always quick to help her when he could. But you needn't worry about her knocking on *your* door because, as I've said, she died some months ago. I believe her name was Eloise."

What a shitty story. *Stuff like that could happen to anyone, I guess, Farthing knew. Don't take your blessings for granted.*

"And here we are, arrived at last," Cooper

announced, pulling past a sign that read MAGNUS ESTATES - DEED RESTRICTED - 45 & OLDER. The park was no more than half a mile from town, which meant that Farthing would be occupying some time at the pub. At the park's entrance stood a fenced-in area containing clusters of smaller caravan-style trailers, which were evidently were being used for resident storage.

Rows of metal boxes lined each side of the road, most quaintly decorated with garden gnomes, bird baths, and shrubs. "Looks just like my old park," Farthing said, more to himself. "Guess they all do." But there didn't seem to be any neglected units; at least the residents took an interest in where they lived. There were single-wides, double-wides, some with custom additions, and none of the cars in the driveways were rattle-traps—always a good sign.

"It's a well-kempt park," Cooper informed. "Quiet, neat as a pin. And not a single crime of note has ever been reported here."

Farthing could've laughed aloud. There'd been *murders* at his own park—mainly old men finally getting sick of their nagging wives and dispatching them—and also a burglary or two (though Farthing pitied the burglar who broke into *his trailer. He had nothing to steal).*

Persons, mostly the elderly, were out for walks, and all paused to cast the Bentley a glance. Farthing waved to one woman but received nothing for the gesture but a blank stare. Cooper drove by First Street, then Second, then Third, and turned on Fourth.

And at the terminus of Fourth Street stood a much more elaborately appointed unit than any he'd seen thus far. It was a double-wide, gleaming and startlingly white, with black trim. It sat perched atop a stout foundation of white-painted cinderblocks, much higher than usual. Clean black shutters sided each window, and they were *real* windows, not the typical hand-crank louvered windows so common. Farthing could never have conceived of owning a trailer so posh and neat. *This thing Is MINE?* Unless there was more fine print, he knew just then that he'd be moving in.

"A rather nice trailer, as far as trailers go, wouldn't you say?" Cooper said after he parked under the portico.

"I love it already," Farthing murmured, still gazing.

"And now?" Cooper popped the Bentley's trunk. "I'd be delighted to give you the twenty-five pence tour."

They got out of the car, and Cooper fetched

Farthing's single suitcase. Around the side, Farthing noticed an entrance to a garden area, this surrounded by a six-foot cinderblock wall; Farthing *hated* seeing neighbors anytime he happened to look out a window. As he mounted the higher than usual front steps, a glance down the street showed him more pedestrians seeming to take an interest at his arrival. *More old people, he saw. Just like me.*

Farthing's worn-out knees ached by the time he'd ascended the short steps. But at once he noticed the door knocker, and an *odd knocker it was. It was a small oval of old dull brass which took the shape of a face. But the face was bereft of features, save for two wide, empty eyes. There was no mouth, no nose, no jawline really—just the eyes. What an UGLY-ass door knocker …*

Cooper jangled keys at the next white paneled front door. "But before we venture in, sir, I'd be negligent not to alert you to the fact that your dear uncle—a marvelous man in myriad ways—did have a disposition to take a pipe on occasion—"

"Take a *pipe?*" Farthing asked quizzically. "Oh, you mean a smoking pipe—"

"Correct, sir—"

"Not that medical marijuana stuff, I hope. You can't go anywhere in America now without smelling that shit. The bus, the grocery store, the laundromat. I even smelled it in the dentist's office recently. It's everywhere now. America's a *nation* of pot-heads. When the Chinese invade us, everyone will be too high to care."

The remark seemed to hector Cooper's train of thought. "No, I'm not referring to marijuana, Mr. Farthing, but instead tobacco, and *bad* tobacco at that. Hence, I'm afraid the trailer's interior might be offensive to your, shall we say, olfactory capabilities."

Farthing had smoked cigarettes in his own trailer for decades, cessating the habit only when his doctor assured him that continuing would relocate him "south of dirt" in short order. "Lead on, Mr. Cooper. I'm sure I've smelled far worse things than lousy pipe smoke."

The door swung open to darkness that seemed foreboding until Cooper's hand patted on a light. The rank air indeed hit Farthing like a blow to the face: dense mustiness tinged with remnant smoke that must now, after so much time, have become imbued into the walls, ceiling, and carpeted floor. *So what?* Farthing considered. *I'll get some air freshener.*

Cooper waded through semi-darkness inside to switch on more lights. Heavy drapes, dark carpets, plush furniture in good repair, and dark paneling comprised the interior's essential outfitting. A spacious living room—complete with a large flat-screen TV—connected to an open kitchen took up the front of the unit, and Farthing was pleased to notice new appliances—quite the opposite of what he had at his own trailer. A narrow hall led down to the bedrooms, the master of which possessed impressive antique furniture, a wonderful old scroll-top desk with letter slots, and a heavily framed four-poster bed. Such was the tale of the interior.

Cooper opened a set of double-doors to expose a lovely view of the back garden bisected by a cement sidewalk and partitions of crushed gravel. There was a quaint glass table and umbrella, cast metal chairs with cushions. What he'd stepped out onto was an elevated porch surrounded by hanging flower pots. But what most arrested Farthing's intrigue was the outdoor patio area.

"What a great-looking place. You won't find anything like that patio in my trailer park back home."

Cooper clearly was happy about the pleasure Farthing was taking thus far in his examination of the property. "Your uncle would be delighted by your approval. But if you'd like to take a turn down to the patio, I'm afraid we must go out the way we came."

"Oh, that's all right—I've got plenty of time to check it out, and the garden too. I guess Uncle Eldred was what you'd call a great gardener."

"Ah, to be sure, gardening was one of his few serious interests. Of course, it could use some pruning and cleaning up, as there's been no one to do that since—well, you know …"

"Sure, but I'm not exactly busy these days," Farthing laughed. Sprucing up the garden would be a delicious occupation for winter.

Next, he noticed a white cement bird bath on a pedestal, but down farther toward the rear cinderblock wall stood another such pedestal, on which sat an object less ordinary: a shining brass sphere, akin to the size of a basketball. "What's that there?"

"Ah, yes, the globe," Cooper began with what seemed a bit of hesitancy. "As I've said, your uncle and I were close friends, and one time not long ago, he expressed his wish to me that upon his demise, he be cremated and that the remnants of his physical body be deposited into that same globe, to rest there in the garden of his property."

Farthing stared at the globe. It gleamed fiercely in the high sun. "So you mean his ashes are in it."

"That's correct, Mr. Farthing, and let me assure

you that the globe's placement here is in no way a provision of your inheritance. In other words, if the situation seems too morbid to you, you're free to dispose of your uncle's remains any way you see fit. After all, we can't say with any certainty, can we, that God cares where our mortal coils are bestowed?"

"I wouldn't dream of disposing of them," Farthing said at once. "If it's what Uncle Eldred wanted, then it's fine by me. In fact, I *like* the idea of some aspect of him being here with me."

"How absolutely grand! I'm thrilled to learn that that's your opinion, and I'm sure Eldred would be too. And now … shall we move our little excursion back inside?"

Farthing followed Cooper back inside, out of the master bedroom, and into the narrow hall, which sported several more closed doors. Behind the first door seemed to be a modest guest bedroom with a single bed, while most of the rest of the room was devoted to high bookshelves.

"Your uncle's library, of which I had occasion to previously mention. Are you much of a reader? Because if that be the case, you've landed in the right place."

Farthing was definitely *not* much of a reader. "Uh …"

"Myself? I've always taken delight in English literature, and if you ask me, there's not a better way to end a day than a good hour's reading before bedtime."

Farthing made a parsimonious nod. "Yes, and I'll definitely check these books out further, later," but yet he knew he'd likely do no such thing. He hadn't read a book in ages. *Well, if I decide to live here,* he thought, *this is one room I'll be using for storage.*

To the next room then, a spacious newly-fitted bathroom and a large shower with handholds; these latter much appreciated by Farthing and his bad balance and bad knees. Back home? Farthing's shower might pass for a telephone booth.

"Fantastic," he said, eyes wide as he looked around.

Several other doors were closets, and in one, on the top shelf, sat an old Polaroid camera, one from the old days, which Farthing remembered from his childhood. The lower shelves were tenanted by a number of other, newer Polaroids. But as Farthing recalled, Polaroid went out of business years ago.

"What you see there, Mr. Farthing," announced Cooper, "is another arm of your uncle's interests."

"Polaroid cameras?" The one on top was one of those fold-up jobs, with parts of it actually made of wood. The lens mount at the front was attached to an accordion-type housing. Folded up, it might be six-by-eight inches, and three thick.

"Yes, but not just that. The camera you see on the top shelf, sir, is the very first model released to the public: The Type 95. They were made available to the American consumer shortly after the end of World War Two. This specimen is likely worth thousands, due to its pristine condition."

The only thing Farthing cared less about than books was photography. "So, a camera buff … Every man needs a hobby, I guess."

"It wasn't so much an interest in cameras or photography but instead an interest in—how shall I put it?—antique implements."

Farthing took that to mean old junk.

"You'll get a better idea in the next, the last room," and Cooper pushed open the door at the end of the hall.

Farthing's brow furrowed upon entrance. First, no window could be detected, which seemed odd since this room made for the very back end of the mobile home. Second, the room stood all but empty. One dim overhead light threw bleary illumination about, and what color the walls were was next to impossible to discern. *What the hell kind of room is this?* he wondered. At the room's rear, a folding metal chair leaned against the wall, and everything before it was just empty carpeted space, save for one bulky single item at the front of the room, maybe five feet high and covered by a brown sheet.

"Voila!" said Cooper in an appropriate flourish. He pulled off the sheet.

There, sitting atop some manner of wooden stand, was a very old television with a round picture tube. "I see," Farthing acknowledged. "My uncle's 'antique implements,' I suppose."

"Yes, and if you're interested in the history of old things, this is one of the very first. There's a date somewhere on the back, your uncle once told me, that says 1940."

Farthing's eyes narrowed. *Did television even exist back them?*

But Cooper answered the thought with immediacy. "Which means this set must be a prototype because televisions evidently weren't available to the public until about 1950. There was very little programming then, and the sets were only affordable to the very rich."

Farthing did his best to feign interest, but he was chiefly wondering if the old set would be too heavy for him to carry out to the garbage himself. "That's fascinating, Mr. Cooper, but I would think that a man with an interest in antiques—especially a financially well-off man—I'd think that he'd have this entire room full of such stuff."

"Well, sir, now that I reflect upon your observation, I must say I that join you in this assessment, and I recognize your point. An old TV, and some old cameras, and some old books, and that's the long and short of it, I'm afraid."

"Does it even work? The television, I mean?" Farthing walked over and looked behind the set. Nothing whatever resembling an antenna jack was evidence.

"Mr. Farthing, if I were to claim sufficient knowledge to answer your question, I'm afraid I'd merely be deceiving you."

"I'm no expert on these things," Farthing said, peering at the TV, "but I'd always heard that analogue television signals stopped broadcasting some time back. To use an old analogue TV like this would require a digital antenna and tuner or something like that. I remember buying one myself about ten years ago."

"And I can ascertain, sir, that you're much better versed on the subject than am I. The armory of my knowledge of such matters, you could say, exists in a state of utter depletion. It seems to me, however, that there is a simple expedient to inform us if the set it is working order …"

"Why didn't I think of that!" Farthing laughed, and he turned on the set.

His efforts were not sufficiently rewarded. Nothing happened, and not even a trace of airwaves fuzz came onto the screen.

"Ah, and there, sir, is the answer to the conundrum," Cooper said.

"Right. Tell me, Mr. Cooper, *what* day is garbage day here?"

Cooper laughed heartily. "Wednesday morn, I do believe." Cooper's portly form led Farthing back to the living room. "But I wouldn't consign it to the rubbish heap just yet. Something that old might indeed be worth a pretty penny to a collector."

Or it might NOT be, Farthing thought. "Thanks for the tour, Mr. Cooper."

"My pleasure, sir. And tonight, may you sleep the sleep of the just." Cooper looked at his watch. "You've my number, call any time with any questions or concerns. I hope your little stay in our town is a fruitful one; in fact, I hope it's a permanent one. Do let me know your decision, once you've made it."

"I definitely will. Thank you, Mr. Cooper."

"And now, the missus is expecting me, and I

wouldn't want to rankle her. Have a wonderful first night in Burnstow!"

The two men shook hands, and Cooper was off.

But Farthing had already made up his mind—with a comparatively light heart—that Burnstow was a place in which he could be happy, and the trailer and other provisions of Uncle Eldred's will would furnish him with more than he would ever need this side of the grave.

Fuck America. He beamed at the thought as he looked around. *This is home.*

At any rate, Mal, given some of her own fucked up proclivities, had found her professional calling (among other things), and here we find her tending to her current client, whose name was as unimportant as his existence as a member of the human species. But first, shall we have a more defined glimpse of Mal herself?

Striking right off the bat was her hair, just short of shoulder-length and eye-catchingly vibrant in its multicolored streaks, which somehow appeared metallic: pink, blue, green, orange, and yellow. She stood average height, slender yet curvy, and possessed of a very low body fat index. She was muscular without appearing masculine; her flat stomach revealed wraiths of washboard abs, and her arms and legs were well-toned. Overall, she exuded a naughty sexuality, and she knew it. A client had paid a tidy sum for laser-removal of all her pubic and underarm hair, and what blossomed from her chest were two tight tangerine-sized breasts with nipples sticking out like golf cleats. Several curious tattoos adorned the lean, nearly flawless physique. Sprouting just a half-inch above the apex of her vulva were two black bat wings that unfolded out to the fronts of her hipbones. A tiny, well-crafted serpent encircled her slit-like bellybutton. She was the living acme of male sex-fantasies.

Mal did work out on occasion but not enough to account for the awesome body. Instead, when reckoned up, it was likely that good genes accounted the most of this superior physicality. But as for her *psychological* makeup, those good genes had missed the mark. More on that, perhaps, later.

"You disgusting little dweeb," she said down to her client. He looked like an accountant, and probably was, balding, skinny, with a long geek neck and Adam's apple sticking out, and he looked ridiculous all trussed up from head to toe in the black rubber suit while the suit was strapped down to the table. The only flesh of his body that showed were his genitals, emerging from an aperture in the rubber.

"For pity's sake," Mal said, grinning at it. "That looks like a penis, only much smaller. Like a little teeny *baby penis. Fuck, my sister's kid had a bigger cock than you the day he was fuckin' born,* you useless little shit."

The client was sort of vibrating in the skin-tight rubber suit. Communicating was difficult because he was wearing a very curious black rubber mask that fit completely over his head. Two black flaps covered his eyes, and there was a black plastic tube (about the width of a toilet paper tube) attached to the mask around his mouth. It stuck up in the manner of a snorkel. She—

smack!

—laid her open palm hard against his exposed testicles.

The groaning that came out of that mouth-tube was priceless and only sounded partly human. The client shuddered on the table.

"Wow, you really are fucked up in the head," she commented, looking down at the man's groin. His penis had turned fully erect. "You twisted fucks are off your trolley. I smack ya in the balls hard as I can, and you pull a boner. What the *fuck is wrong with you? Your daddy must* 'a dropped you on your head when you were little. Fucked up your brain." She—

smack!

—smacked his balls again, if anything, harder than the first time. Now, he was almost convulsing on the table, and this time, his moan sounded like a cow lowing.

"I'll have to record that and use it for my ringtone," she said. "And would you look at that?" She gave his cock a few strokes. "Fuckin' thing's even harder now, you whack-job. Well, fuck it then, I guess it's time to start this loser party," and then she slopped some baby oil on his erection and started jerking it. "You like that, fuck-face? Hmm? Yeah, I'll bet you do. Let's see if this micro-penis is good for anything, you pathetic wanker. I'll bet you're thinkin' 'bout your daddy, hmm? About when you were a baby and your daddy jerked off in your mouth three times a day 'cos he was so poor he couldn't even afford baby food? Hmm?"

The baby-food line always did it. The client squirmed in the suit, ejaculating numerous spurts up onto his chest. When the spasms ended—

smack!

—she slapped his balls hard one more time.

"No wonder you're not married," she made the observation. "You didn't last ten seconds. But it's all for the best, I suppose. A sick, pathetic loser like you shouldn't be allowed to reproduce. We've got enough useless perverted *fucks* in this world. We sure don't need any more."

She looked at the clock. *Thank God it's almost done.* "Yum-Yum Time, little baby," she cooed. With a plastic spoon, she scooped the semen up off his chest and dropped each spoonful into the plastic mouth-tube. "And you swallow it, you little bitch, or else this will happen," and she put her palm over the tube's opening, sealing off his air. "Go on, swallow like a good little baby."

He was jerking in place, mewling now, unable to breathe.

"Swallow—"

Then that big Adam's apple moved under the rubber, and she took her hand off. "Good, good boy! How's your own nut taste, your little puke? And don't worry, we're not done yet." She dragged over a plastic cereal bowl, only there was no cereal in it. "Got to make sure the customer gets his money's worth, don't we?"

The bowl had half a dozen used condoms in it that the other girls in the shop had been all too happy to contribute.

She turned each one upside-down and emptied them into the mouth-tube. But when she looked into the tube, she saw the pile of pearlescent slop just sitting there. First, she grabbed his Adam's apple and squeezed so hard his butt came off the table. "You suck that shit down and swallow it, motherfucker"—then she pressed her palm back over the top of the tube—"or I will do the world a *big* favor and just fuckin' KILL you right here and now! You hear me, little baby? Walking shit like you does not deserve to live! Now swallow!"

Now he was trembling on the table and making some shrill, very disturbing noises in his throat. She heard the gulp and smiled as she envisioned all that dirty john cum sliding down into the fucker's stomach, but she kept her hand on the tube a while longer. *Careful careful. I don't want to have to get rid of a body tonight …*

She'd gotten rid of a few in her time, but that was another story.

He wheezed like a sucking chest wound when she took her hand off the tube, but before he could get his breath back—-

kurrrr-HOCK

—she dragged up a formidable wad of phlegm and spat it down the tube.

"That's the chaser." She pulled the eye-patches off his mask and waved bye-bye. "Toodles, lover. See ya next week." She turned to walk out but

55

then—

smack!

—whacked her open palm against his balls one last time. It made a crack like one of those stropping belts barbers used to use. "Fooled ya!" She giggled. She walked out.

Just giving him what he paid for, she thought. *The SICK FUCK.*

In the break room, Savva sat with one leg all the way back behind her shoulder; she was putting in a diaphragm. "How'd yours go?"

"Oh, fabulous, easiest john I've ever had, and he pays five hundred each time. Barely get my hands dirty, and it's kind of fun feedin' the arsehole a big rasher of other blokes' cum. And every time I crack him in the balls, he gets harder. I just don't get it."

"Me either, love. Men just ain't right. Like me next one."

"Who?" Mal asked.

"The ca-ca guy. Pays me three to shit on his cock while he jerks off."

Mal winced. "Fuck that shit."

Savva chuckled. "He kind of does. And he looks kind of like the old Prime Minister."

"Don't I wish that trainwreck would walk in here someday."

Savva pointed to the room Mal just left. "Aren't

you gonna let him up?"

"Oh, no, I always wait ten or fifteen minutes. Give the shit-head time to sweat."

"You choke him too?"

"Oh, fuck yes. One time he came just from that, can ya believe it? I do anything he wants—well, almost anything. He keeps begging me to piss in the breathing tube—"

"Oh, I would *love* to do that!" Savva exclaimed.

"Yeah, well, ya gotta be careful with that kind of shit. If he doesn't swallow the piss fast enough, the fucker could drown." Mal smiled wistfully. "Can't you imagine that? Drowning a bloke in his own piss?"

"Makes me soak just thinking about it. All these fuckin' arseholes. They're just total shit."

Bunky, the six-foot-nine bouncer, stuck his head in and patted the wall. "Mal? Phone call, hon."

Mal stood up. "It's probably that office manager from Highgate. His daughter got killed in a car wreck last year, and he pays me to put on her clothes and act dead while he fucks me."

Savva just shook her head. "Like what I just told ya, they're all just total shit …"

Mal slipped into the office. Bunky sat at the desk, his big legs spread. He wore a shabby suit and tie yet fancied he looked like a high-end gangster. He slid the phone across the desk, and Mal picked it up.

"Mal here."

In an instant, her eyes widened, and she came alert almost like a soldier coming to the position of attention. "I see," she said.

A pause.

"Yes," she said.

Another pause.

"Yes, sir. I'll be there in the morning," and then she hung up.

"Be where in the mornin', little miss?" Bunky demanded.

She couldn't say no; the money was just too good. "What's it to you?"

"What's it to me? I run this place, ya tart!"

"No, Nick runs this place, you answer the phone and clean the pisser."

Bunky scowled. "So where might you be headin' off to then?"

"A nice little town east of here. You may have heard of it. It's called None 'a Your Bloody Business."

"Fuck that, Mal! Didn't you just have time off a couple 'a months ago?"

Mal began to dress, covering up those firm tangerine-sized breasts and plump nipples. "Yeah.

'T'was a free country last time I looked, Bunky."

"Is it now? Well, Nick ain't gonna like it, young lady."

"Oh, well then tell Nick he can fire me, which he *won't* do 'cos I bring more money into this outhouse than all the other birds combined." This was quite true, and she wasn't worried about her boss. She grabbed her keys from her purse.

"Well, when ya comin' back?" Bunky demanded,

"When I get back." She headed for the door.

"Well, hold up there, love. Since you'll be away a while"—he opened his pants and pulled out his penis and balls—"how's about a quick blow job? You know. Just for the hell of it?"

She looked at him, looked at his genitals, then said, "I'd rather defecate out my mouth," and left the shop.

Once Farthing set himself down with a beer from Uncle Eldred's fridge, he sluggishly prepared a To Do List, now that he'd decided to say. Essentially, all of his friends back in the States were now dead, which made severing ties all the easier. *What about mail forwarding? he wondered, and what about the hellish IRS?* These were nuisances he'd have to look into quickly. And he'd have to inquire at the Burnstow bank if any manner of reciprocity existed between it and American banks, and how to transfer his Social Security to his British account. *What a fuckin' pain in the ass … but it can't be THAT hard.* People expatriated all the time without officially terminating their citizenship. And with that, Farthing's desultory habits took hold, and he resolved to pursue these matters tomorrow.

Or the next day.

Connecting his laptop to the local internet proved easy once he located the router box. The TV remote sat right on the sofa arm, but he left it for now. There'd be plenty of time to compare British TV to American; he could only suspect the two were similar and loaded mostly with shows and movies too insipid for his liking: lame comedy and implausible thrillers. No, now a more detailed tour seemed in order, a closer inspection of the advantages of his property.

He got up and moseyed about the living room. A six-sided mirror hung head-high near the door, and farther off was a painting of an old town; tiny letters identified it as Bury St. Edmunds. *What kind of a name is that for a town?* And then a harder squint showed him a hill behind the town that seemed to be a place for gibbets complete with bodies hanging by the neck. *What happened to Home*

Sweet Home, and shit like that? These Brits were morbid. Was this town nearby? Were people really executed here long ago? *Cheerio, my ass …*

He wandered about more; his beer was good but strong. Mid-sip, he stopped, astonished, because facing him, near the entrance to the hall, was a curio rack on which stood a framed eight-by-ten photograph. *That HAS to be Uncle Eldred,* came the realization. It was a portrait shot of a man who looked quite similar to Farthing; the man in the photo appeared to be around Farthing's age now. Large eyes, an earnest smile, and trimmed beard were the salient features. *So there you are, Uncle Eldred! How's it going?*

Next, and without forethought, Farthing exited the front door and walked around to the back garden. Birds chirped at him from the high cinderblock fence. *They're probably pissed. I'll have to fill the bird bath.* Though overgrown, the garden planters were full of bright, hardy flowers, and the fragrance couldn't have been more pleasant. But this rear area was larger than he'd thought; it was almost as though it had been lain out with a view to mislead, for he couldn't at first find the brass globe which he'd seen from the bedroom balcony, but—

There it was, hidden by some standing bushes.

61

Farthing watched his own distorted reflection as he approached it—

Whoa!

A breath caught in his chest. For the briefest moment, the edges of his vision not only detected his own warped reflection but also that of something else. He turned with a start and laughed. Of course, it was nothing but a shifting tree branch or something of the kind. *I'm getting skittish in my old age …*

He refaced the globe, almost blinded by the sun's high glare. "Hello, Uncle Eldred. I dearly wish I could've met you. Thank you for leaving me your home and the rest." He laid his opened palm atop the globe—daintily, for he expected it to be fiercely hot from the sunlight. However, if anything, it was cool to the touch. He altered the angle by which he looked at the globe, changing his perspective away from the glare, and he noticed some faint engravings, he thought. Were they words or pictures? But another moment's scrutiny told him it was both.

First, a simple etching of two open eyes. Below this, the words *Pater Terrae, Per Me Vide Terrum.* This flustered Farthing. He'd failed Latin in eleventh grade and had no wish to return to it, and as he didn't have a pen or sheet of paper with him, he promised himself he'd copy the words down another time to have them translated, knowing full well the true likelihood of that was near nil.

All at once, the day's heat was just becoming oppressive. "Until next time, Uncle," he bid the globe. "Have a pleasant day," and then he walked back to the front. He was just tall enough to glimpse over the top of the cinderblock fence.

A black car rumbled by, a very sleek looking one, like a ritzy sports car. It seemed to slow down as it was passing Farthing's unit, and he immediately went up on tiptoes for a better look.

Farthing didn't know from cars, but he wasn't stupid; what rumbled just before his property *had* to be something very expensive. It looked futuristic. The dark-tinted glass prevented him from noting anything about the driver, which made him angry. What was the car doing just sitting there? Farthing got the unpleasant impression that the unseen driver was staring at him, and not in any way that could be thought of as positive. *Rude motherfucker,* he thought, and then rushed beyond the fence and strode toward the rumbling car.

It drove off at once.

"That's not something you see every day, eh?" a woman's cockney voice came from somewhere. There was something sexy and lilting about how it carried the accent. "At least not in a trailer court. That was a brand-new Lamborghini!"

The surprise voice distracted him. "A Lam—Oh, wow. How do you like that?" He looked over at the woman, shapely if a bit rag-tag in baggy shorts, flip-flops, and some kind of spandex-type shirt. She had long brown hair down to her waist, and as she walked, she had two plastic shopping bags dangling from her hands. By the time Farthing thought to introduce himself, she was too far down the road. Several cats frolicked behind her.

Must be Cooper's Cat Lady. And he's right, she's not too hard on the eyes. Farthing felt slightly ashamed staring after her, but only slightly. *That's some backside, he thought. Wouldn't mind seeing her in her birthday suit …*

And it was either ironic or exceedingly coincidental, but in a very short time, Farthing would do just that.

He went back into the trailer, relishing the air-conditioning, and walked around some more, looking things over. The back room was where he found himself first, before the ancient television. When he tried turning it on again, there was still nothing—not even that *pop,* not that crackling sound of the tube just getting juice. He pulled it out a little and examined the back.

Of all the fucked up …

His original intention was to make sure the TV was plugged in. It was not.

Nor was there even an outlet in the wall anywhere behind it. And on top of that—

Farthing patted around the back to make sure his eyes weren't deceiving him.

Even if there *had* been an outlet in the wall to plug the set into, there was no plug, no power cord whatever coming out of the TV. And there was no coaxial hook-up, of course, nor was there even a screw-fitted connector for an antenna.

How the FUCK can this thing work if there's no power cord?

It was ridiculous, and he continued to inspect all sides of the set impatiently, as was his wont. Absolutely nothing existed on the back, save for the protrudement found on any cathode-tube television.

This dumbass thing is headed straight for the garbage, but … some OTHER day.

Another minute found him in the spare bedroom that also housed his uncle's bookshelves. He scanned some titles listlessly. *A Parable Of This Unhappy Condition,* read one. Then, *A Defence of Episcopacy* by the Rev. John Benwell Haynes. Then, *The Life And Times Of Canon Alberic de*

Mauleon. Farthing couldn't conceive of books more unreadable nor more boring than the likes of these, and that's where his perusal came to a halt. But—

What have we here?

On the lowest shelf sat something like a fat photo album. Farthing drew it out at once. Perhaps here he might find more photos of his uncle as well as other relatives of which he was unaware.

And perhaps he would find nothing of the sort.

Holy shit! Now I know what Eldred was doing with those Polaroids, the old dog!

Farthing was actually giddy with bemusement; he rushed into the living room's better light, flumped onto the couch, and slowly scanned the album's first pages. They were all loaded with Polaroids of nude women. And this next one, with very long brunette hair, could only be the Cat Lady whom he'd just seen walking home with groceries, though this picture had to have been snapped over twenty years ago. *Buck-ass naked, he thought, the dirty girl!* If a photo could be described as *loud,* this was it.

The woman sat spread-eagled on a couch—the same couch, in fact, that Farthing now occupied—her pelvis lewdly thrust forward. This deliberate pose made no secret of the pink folds of her sex, pushed out from the nest of abundant pubic hair.

The tip of her index finger looked pressed into the nub of the clitoris. But more paramount than that were the magnificent bare breasts—double-Ds, for sure—with nipples sticking out like pink cabinet knobs. Farthing could've howled at an adjoining photo, which depicted the same woman from mid-thigh to neck, lying with arched back. Even this non-digital photo technology was sharp enough for Farthing to easily see foot-long gouts of semen spread over her belly and chest.

That HAS to be Uncle Eldred's spooge, he realized. *Good for you, Uncle! That's really hosing her down!*

Farthing noticed now, with some accelerated excitement, just how *fat* the album was, and the voyeur in him actually admitted that this was about the most interesting thing to happen to him in a long time. Each page proffered several new ladies, nearly all of them naked and nearly all of them trampishly attractive. *This is like Hustler in the old days, Farthing thought. The album clearly demonstrated that Uncle Eldred was all-inclusive with regard to his tastes. Women of all shapes and sizes had posed for his uncle's camera, from petite to full-figured, small-breasts to huge-breasted, tall and short. There were several stills of each girl, and quite often one still was devoted to a display of Eldred's semen spattered on some part of the woman's body. One split-beaver after the next,* he thought.

Such was the curse of a great many solitary men no longer touched by vestiges of younger days. Farthing was *enthralled by this album. It seemed so much more interesting than typical internet porn; it seemed more real because the women had availed their nudity to Uncle Eldred in this very room. Eldred sure knew how to let the good times roll …* With more than a few of the girls, there was a side-shot photo of her mouth in the unhesitant process of fellatio, and the penis also displayed could only be Uncle Eldred's. *Homemade smut doesn't get better than this, Farthing concluded.*

The enthusiasm triggered by the album's discovery occluded Farthing's acknowledgment that his life was and always had been especially dull and unfulfilled. But such things like this gave him a bit of a spark that he found invigorating. The delicious images—dozens and dozens of them—made him lose track of time. Each time he decided to put the album away, the next girl insisted that he keep his eyes in attendance. One after another. Each rise of the next cardboard page made his heart race and stiffened him below the belt to a degree he'd thought was lost to him. At about the middle of the book, he even found Bernice, the barmaid. Only much younger. She offered a vulpine grin, displaying an hourglass figure as her hands hoisted up mammoth breasts. The next photo showed a spent cock lying limp against said breasts, having liberally dispersed its seminal wares all over the mammarian landscape. *Damn, Uncle Eldred!* Farthing thought. *You're a regular porn star …*

Farthing spent little time wondering just who these women were in the scheme of things. Prostitutes, of course, all with an eye for the accommodating old rich guy. Farthing grinned over at Eldred's framed photo. *More power to ya, Uncle Eldred …*

When the album finally released his attentions, he saw that it was nine p.m. That's how engrossed Farthing had been. The entire day had elapsed, and now it was nighttime, with his face buried in these fascinatingly lewd images. He slipped the book beneath the coffee table (for later consultation, no doubt). It was getting late, yes, but not too late for a nightcap at the bar.

The chorus of crickets throbbed pleasantly as Farthing left his trailer. It was a bright moonlight night; an owl hooted in the distance. The trailer park extended in tranquil solitude—this was quite a difference from his park in Florida. Rows of trailers extended down the road, with windows warmly lit. Pin-drop silent. But as he walked down Fourth Street, a sleek-looking car idled by, turned, and headed the opposite direction. Farthing noticed the word Ferrari on the back; moreover, when it traversed the street completely, it seemed to slow, then stop right in front of his trailer.

What the fuck is all this sports car shit going on here? Cars like that cost a fortune, just like Lamborghinis. Farthing remained where he stood, staring back. Eventually, the car pulled away and disappeared.

A ten-minute leisurely walk took him into town and into the Mattshaw Pub. A few cars were parked out front, and a little music could be heard, along with soft bar talk. No one so much as looked at him when he entered; several patrons sat about at various tables.

"Welcome back, Mr. Farthing!" Bernice greeted from behind the almost empty bar.

Farthing pulled up a stool, at once feeling better connected to his roots. "Hi, Bernice. You couldn't keep me away. I'd like a pint of … whatever you served me earlier." He found her all the more interesting now that he'd seen the nude picture of her; it didn't matter how long ago it had been taken. This bid a multitude of questions he could not ask, however. *Damn, what a body she had,* he thought, watching the swell of her bosom as she poured the beer. *And it's still not bad now ...* He turned his gaze away quickly; he didn't want to be caught staring.

A glance around the bar showed him nondescript patrons, all male, all older. One man, at least, assured Farthing he wasn't the oldest person here: a gray-haired, stoic-faced man, neatly dressed, with owlish round eyeglasses. He was bent over, writing in a pad.

Bernice set down his own beer. "I see you've taken note of our Professor Oldys. Nice enough chap, I suppose. That man come in 'ere every night for *years,* swallow hisself three pints 'n' scribble in his pad and don't leave but a pitiful couple of shillings for tip." She huffed a laugh. "You know what they say about us Brits, eh? Ain't no bigger tight-wads on Earth ... except for the bloody Canadians!"

Next, she leaned forward on the bar, making it near impossible for Farthing to ignore the plentitude of her bosom. *Damn ...*

"So how you likin' your Uncle Eldred's place?"

"Well, I'm liking it so much that I've already decided to relocate here permanently. The town's beautiful, it's right near the beach, Brits are much nicer than Americans, and, well, I like your bar a lot and it's walking distance. So that was it for me."

"Well, 'ow wonderful that is! I'd say that calls for a shot on the house to celebrate."

"Why, well, thanks much."

With her back to him now, Farthing was helpless to refrain further visual examination. She had to be into her fifties, but her frame still preserved some welcome curves remnant of the nude photos. *That's a serious caboose on this woman …*

She turned back to him and gave him a shot. "To Mr. Farthing, for choosing England over the US."

"I'll drink to that." Farthing downed the shot. *Bleck! Ouzo!* He tried his best not to gag. "Thank you, Bernice. And you can drop the 'mister.' My parents demonstrated their terrible sense of humor by giving me the first name Icarus. So please just call me Farthing."

"Happy to oblige, Farthing." She'd downed her own shot without a hitch. "Icarus, eh? Weren't that the Greek bloke who—"

"Who flew too close to the sun, yes. But I'm happy to say, that's not a character trait of *mine*."

"Not very daring, are you? Just as well these days. So, 'ave you found anything interesting in your uncle's trailer?"

What to say? Hmm … "Now that you mention it,

today I've noticed not one but two very expensive sports cars driving by the place and giving it a look over, all in the past few hours."

Bernice made a pondering expression. "Guess maybe they ain't heard old Eldred died, huh?"

"They?"

"What like I was tellin' ya earlier," Bernice said, now with her chin in her palm. "Likely it was some 'a them blokes he cronied around with, that travel club or whatever it was he were in. Lotta rich men, they, and a lot of 'em had very expensive cars, especially the forig fellas. McLarens, Ferraris, Rolls."

"Hmm. Yes, I suppose that makes sense."

"'Twas a big deal here in town, it was, that bunch comin' in here with Eldred. All those shiny cars parked out front. Then they'd go back ta Eldred's trailer, and I can't imagine what they was all doin' *there*. Might be able to hazard a guess, though."

Farthing was about to inquire, but she turned around again to wash the two shot glasses, and there his eyes went again, running up the plush curves of her body from behind like intent hands, then he imagined the hands slipping forward to cradle those colossal breasts. Melded into this fantasy was the same woman but younger, the woman in Uncle Eldred's perverse photo album.

The potency of these images proved themselves right away; Farthing got an erection faster than he had in years.

There was a snide grin on her when she turned back around. "Let me guess. You found that bleedin' book, didn't ya?"

"Buh–book?"

"Old Eldred's photo album stuffed full 'a Polaroids of any woman he could pay ta get starkers."

How could she possibly—Farthing felt like a wall had collapsed on him. "Um, I …"

"I seen ya starin' at me couple times already—"

Farthing's face turned red at once. "I wasn't—"

"I could see ya in the reflection," Bernice laughed, pointing to the mirror behind the bar. "Guess you Americans ain't much for the details 'a things. One person ya can't never lie to is a bartender."

Caught dead to rights, Farthing realized. "Um, well, yeah. I confess. Sorry."

"Ain't nothin' to apologize for," she said. "Any woman tell ya she don't like ta be looked at is a liar. But I could see your brain tickin' away, thinkin', 'Well I'll be, this is the same bird I seen naked in Uncle's photo album.' That old perv, but weren't none of us complainin' 'cos that man, he paid righteous. Lotta folks make judgments about stuff like that, but what no man realize is how much harder it is for a woman to make it in this world."

He could only hope his face wasn't still the color of a tomato. "I believe that very much, Bernice. I was just … taken by surprise is all."

"I'll bet you was. Bet there's at least a hundred different women in that album, goin' way, way back, probably to the fifties, it wouldn't surprise me none."

"It's odd, though," Farthing thought to add. "Obviously, my uncle had this vice—pornography—but he also had money, so why not use better cameras, with better resolution? Better pictures?"

"A odd card, he was. But it was old things he liked best of all, like those shitty old Polaroid cameras, and not even new ones. 'Old is always better than new,' he used ta say." She chuckled. "And I don't think he fancied the idea of anyone workin' at the photomat seein' his collection. Guess you also saw that nutty cat lady in the album too."

"Why, yes, I did, just after seeing her in real life bringing home groceries."

"She were a wild one in 'er day, I'll tell ya. Did more 'n' my share of doubles with her."

Doubles? Farthing wondered. He doubted she meant tennis. "What do you mean, doubles?"

She refilled his glass as she chuckled. "Don't get out much, do ya, Farthing? See, we all loved your uncle on account of the liberality he had with his wallet. All the women in that photo album? We was all doin' more than just posin' for pictures."

This was something he'd already considered in general *Bernice just straight-out admitted that she'd been a prostitute in the past, and one of her 'johns' was Uncle Eldred.*

This was getting uncomfortable, so he excused himself for the GENTS. Grafitti-less, clean, and no rubber machines, unlike most bar men's rooms in Florida. *My first piss in a foreign country;* the thought amused him. When he went back out, he noticed the professor leaving with his folded-up newspaper.

"Do I remember you sayin'," Bernice began when he was back on his stool, "that you never once met your uncle, nor seen a picture of him?"

"That's correct, odd as it seems. But I always sent him a card for Christmas and his birthday; my parents insisted. In fact, they always suggested that I might one day be rewarded for the kindness, and now I see that I have. He left everything to me."

"And speakin' of birthdays, I'll likely never forget his. July thirty-first—"

"That's right! But why would you remember that?"

"Two reasons. One, every birthday, he come in 'ere and drink his arse off, pay everyone's tab, and tip *big*—not like that skin-flint professor just left."

Stop staring at her tits! Farthing ordered himself. *Stop it!* Had they actually gotten bigger since he'd returned from the bathroom? "You said two reasons. What's the second?"

"July thirty-first is an olden time holiday for certain places in England. It's called Lammas Eve, and it goes back to the time before Christianity got here solid. To regular folk, it celebrated the first bread of the harvest, and they had what they called a Loaf Mass, thankin' God for a good bounty. Ah, but there was other folks who take it a bit different, the Loaf Mass, that is. See, it weren't God they worshiped but the Devil, and their turn at the Loaf Mass was pluckin' a innocent virgin, rapin' 'er six ways to Sunday, and then they bury her alive at sundown; but, see, what they bury with her is a loaf 'a bread made from the first wheat. And all the night long they have theirselfs a *orgy*, they did, and the following sundown they dig up that poor dead girl, and they break that loaf 'a bread and eat it, sort of thankin' the Devil for his protection. Some even say they'd rape the dead girl too, to offend

God, but I don't know as I believe all *that*."

Wow, Farthing reasoned. *These British have been FUCKED UP in their time.*

"Yeah, your uncle, he always have hisself a good time with *that*—his birthday, I mean. Always jokin' how his blood come down from a long line 'a heretics and warlocks. He'd say all the best warlocks was born on occult holidays, but a'course he were joking." Then Bernice caught Farthing looking right at her bosom, smiled traceably, but neglected to mention it. "So, Farthing, when might *your* birthday be?"

"Well, it's not an occult holiday, I can tell you that," he reflected. "It's February first."

Bernice gave a loud hoot at that. "I'll have you know, February first is Candlemas Eve, and there ain't many occult holidays bigger 'n' it."

Farthing frowned. "What the hell's Candlemas Eve?"

"Day a'fore Candlemas, what day the early pagans thank their gods for lettin' the winter be halfway over. But over time, it come ta be something else, a time when witches and warlocks call up demons to plague those that persecute their kind." She slapped a hand down on the bartop and laughed. "I'll tell ya, Farthing, you sure picked a doozy of a day to be born on!"

Farthing was not particularly surprised when, walking back home after last call, he realized he'd had too much to drink.

Great. What's that say about you? First night in your new home—a new COUNTRY—and you're shit-faced ...

But the beer and the conversation had been too good. Farthing made the self-assessment that he was allowed to live a little too. And the calm quiet night was a pleasure to be in. Back home, walking home from a bar this late meant that if you were even still alive upon arrival, you'd at least be minus a wallet. The tranquility cocooned him, the weather perfect. The ocean air even revived him a bit, and when he looked out toward the coast, he could see the winking gleam of a dim and murmuring sea.

Eventually, he made it back into his trailer and locked the door behind him. On the couch, he pulled back out the album, was about to re-examine it, when it occurred to him that he hadn't really eaten anything today. *You should've gotten something at the pub, dumbass ...* So he decided to check the kitchen for food, took a deep breath, and promptly flopped over on the couch and fell asleep.

Was he dreaming? He must be.

First, he was standing at the double-doors in Uncle Eldred's bedroom; he was looking through the glass panes at the moonlit rear-yard, right at the globe containing Eldred's ashes. Behind it, half-concealed by the shrubs, stood a slender man in black garb. This being a dream, Farthing went out on the porch to demand an explanation as to this man's presence, but when he got there—to the edge of the porch—he realized that he would be addressing his demand to nothing more than a black wooden post, like something people hung flower pots on. He smiled at his ineptitude.

Wait a minute, he thought in the dream. *This is a dream, isn't it?*

It must be, because in the next moment, he was walking toward a sound—was it a digging sound?—that seemed to issue from the very back of his enclosed yard, but as he ventured there, the setting of the dream changed, as sometimes happens in dreams, and he received the impression that he was still in the same place and then again wasn't.

It was no sedate backyard that met his gaze now. He was standing in a wooded clearing—at night— and there it was, audibly more pronounced: that digging sound. Farthing seemed to stand there without being noticed by the two woolen-clad men digging. It was nighttime, but the moon was different from when Farthing had last seen it in his backyard; it was a sharp sickle with a few threads of clouds drifting across. In a relatively short period of time, the two men in woolen cloaks slowed their toils, and it was then that Farthing became more keenly—and nauseously—aware of other details of the scene. It was clearly a grave plot the two men were excavating. The area was not just a home for this single grave but countless graves, all evidently very shallow, for the air all around was heavy with the soul-upheaving stench of death.

One of the men said, "Qof fesh, aye?"

The other stopped digging. "Fo shin, aye. Lam ned tof."

Both men dropped their shovels, strange, flat straight-edged things, and reached down, and from the hole, they extracted the sought-after corpse—buried coffinless, wrapped in some manner of sackcloth.

"Gimmel, yue. May Kaf," one said.

All the way out they hauled the wrapped corpse, and made no long work of unrolling the shroud. This act revealed the blanched nude body of a young girl whose head lolled back, showing the wide-open but very dead eyes and an agape mouth. Some lump of some sort sat positioned on the corpse's stomach, and one of the men picked it up. Farthing thought the object must be a loaf of bread.

"May ot bet," the man said. "Yue fok," and then he walked away with the loaf, heading toward what looked to be a group of dwellings far off in the dim night. The second man hoisted up his cloak and knelt down between the corpse's spread legs—

It was at this point that Farthing, now oozing clammy sweat, convulsed vertiginously, and his next awareness was this: he was bent over in his brick-enclosed back yard, projectile vomiting onto an unfortunate row of gardenias. It was not alone the dream-vision he'd just had that triggered this involuntary eruption but also the presiding grave-stench that seemed to follow him back from his dream-location to his very real backyard.

Fuck this, his thoughts muttered. *What's wrong with me?* He stumbled off, ludicrously stamping his feet as if his shoes were crafted of cement. He wended around the front, stumbled up the front steps—almost falling—and barged back into the trailer. Locking the door behind him, he sighed loudly in relief.

Why?

Because he'd felt certain that there'd been something behind him outside, giving chase. *Safe now, he thought. He took one step, and stopped. But still drunk as fuck …*

Here, then, began his trek to Uncle Eldred's bedroom, but he reminded himself, *It's MY bedroom now, since I'm the new master here.* As carefully as possible, he shuffled down the hall, steadying the drunken footfalls by pressing his hands against each side of the wall. But he stopped abruptly, and his heart leapt, for when he glanced down the hall, he saw—

"Who are you!" he yelled.

Was there a slim darkly-dressed man standing at the hall's end? For a moment, it seemed so, but as he stared further, he thought the figure looked more like—well—a black wooden post of some kind, like the one in the garden. He scrunched his face up and violently shook his head. *It's not fuckin' possible, you drunk asshole!* And when he looked again, naturally, the mirage was gone. *See what happens when you drink your face off? You get alcohol poisoning. You begin to hallucinate.* At least the brief scare had sobered him up a bit, but when he continued toward the master bedroom, he stopped yet again.

No darkly dressed man this time, no black

wooden post. Instead, what halted him in his tracks was his noticing a fluttering whitish line of light in the gap of the door at the end of the hall, the room with that old TV set in it. This observation could only mean one thing: the set was turned on.

He opened the door and drifted into the room. Yes, the set was indeed turned on, its strange round screen full of shifting fuzz, but there was no noise, no static sound.

Just utter silence.

He moved slowly to the set and looked behind it. He'd looked for the plug and power cord earlier and found none, but something had obviously escaped his notice. *Missed it,* he thought and then pulled the TV, stand and all, away from the wall.

The same fucked up shit …

As before, no power cord came out of the set, and there was no power socket anywhere on the back wall. There were several such outlets on other walls, but there was nothing plugged into any of them. Farthing just stared at the television's screen full of lit fuzz. For some reason, any sound—just crackling static—would've been less unnerving than the silence.

Okay. That's it for tonight, and Farthing pushed the TV stand back against the wall but—

"Drat! You bitch!"

Something sharp on the back of the set had pricked his finger, and did a good job of it. Furious with himself, he brought his fingertip to his mouth, tasted copper and felt pain more significant than a simple pin prick. He was tempted even to kick the television over. *Fucker!* he thought, still sucking his finger. *Just a big, useless hunk of shit!*

He gazed behind the set to ascertain what had jabbed him but saw nothing. Perhaps it was the point of a screw, or a tiny piece of wire? Still, he saw nothing, and his ire remained because it really hurt, and the tiny puncture on his fingertip still hurt.

And it was still bleeding.

He'd have to find a band-aid. He bent to turn the set off.

But he didn't turn it off.

There was now no shifting fuzz on the screen. In fact, the picture was crystal clear, as sharp as the 4K sets he'd seen in stores. He stroked his chin, peering. He did not immediately cogitate the blaring deviation from logic—that being, how could a television without a power cord possibly be showing *anything on its screen?*

Instead, his attention focused on the broadcast. It had to be some Hollywood dramatization because the details were just too keen. They were staggeringly grim as well. First, Farthing saw a twenty-foot-high pile of severed human heads, all *freshly* severed, and behind that, several more piles extended, each demonstrating descending levels of decomposition. The final pile, in fact, consisted of bare skulls. *Must be some dramatization of one of those African genocides,* Farthing thought. The severed heads were all very dark-skinned, and so were the uniformed soldiers milling about. But if this were a Hollywood dramatization, it seemed ill-proportioned. It was merely the camera roving around the perimeter, betwixt the head-piles, not much in the way of lenscraft; it was almost as though the cameraman were walking around the scene, and there didn't seem to be any cuts yet. Was this just rough footage for some movie about genocide?

Now the camera plunged into jungle until a crowded clearing appeared. More armed soldiers stood idly in a circle, while men in khaki clothes were pinning mostly naked captives to the ground. Tourniquets were then applied near the shoulder of each captive, then—

Farthing had to look away.

The arms of these captives were being severed with machetes, the tourniquets of course staving off blood loss. The wounded captives were then shoved off into the jungle. Many minutes went by like this, and many, many arms were severed and thrown into the back of a truck. Groups of soldiers leaned on their rifles, grinning, smoking cigarettes, as more, still more arms were cut off. The camera moved in on silent screaming faces, and in spite of there being no sound, Farthing thought he could hear the ghost of each *thwack!* each time a machete blade fell to lop off an arm.

Farthing was no history buff nor a news hound, but he thought he recalled hearing of such things back in the '90s. Several genocides had taken place in Africa, usually due to food, politics, and ethno-supremacy, and one place in particular, in Rwanda. Over half a million people were slaughtered, while select captives had their arms cut off, the wounds tied off, and were banished to the jungle. With no arms, they couldn't feed or defend themselves and were doomed to be eaten alive by wild animals. Just another shining example of the wonders of the human race.

Farthing watched with morbid fascination this unlikely "dramatization." Now the soldiers were bayoneting children as they were released from caged trucks; the smaller children were carried off on soldiers' shoulders and dropped into a large high-walled circle, around which stood more soldiers hooting and hollering in silence. In time, the camera veered into the circle to show the children convulsing in horror as several fifteen-foot pythons slowly encircled their soon-to-be prey. It was nauseating, and Farthing, again, looked away when a python lunged, unhinged its jaws, and swallowed whole a naked three- or four-year-old girl. Farthing nearly fainted at the split-second glimpse of the *lump sliding down into the snake's writhing body.*

Finally, then, the scene cut to another place, and the camera was now entering what appeared to be a prison with barred cells on either side and black men jammed into each cell. Soldiers were pushing in wheelbarrows heaped high with steaming human arms, while other gloved soldiers tossed several of the arms into each cell. The inmates wasted no time fighting over the arms and gnawing the meat off them. At least Farthing knew now what the oppressors did with all those arms.

Farthing was dizzy. Deep down, it occurred to him that there was something very wrong about these "dramatizations," but he was not yet ready to consciously admit that. Now the camera's point of view soared away to some other clearing where several dozen naked men and women lay out in a field with wrists and ankles bound. Several large supply trucks pulled into view and began nonchalantly running over the captives, leaving them to quaver and convulse in the dirt, bones broken, organs ruptured. After another break-neck thrust of the camera, a row of ten naked pregnant women were bound to poles, then the camera pulled back to show still more soldiers, these charging their rifles for a firing squad. The commander of the squad dropped his raised hand, all of the rifles bucked, and in utter silence, each bound woman went limp. Several immediately miscarried.

What remained of Farthing's drunkenness disappeared instantly; he was cold-staring sober as he reflected on what he'd just seen. It just looked too real to be dramatization or CGI. Why would a film company fictionalize something like *that, a horrific tragedy that the western world pretty much ignored?*

He knew he couldn't watch this stuff anymore, so he leaned over to turn off the set but noticed the channel knob, or what he presumed was the channel knob because there were no numbers on it. He turned it but found there were no "stops" like the TVs of old that he remembered. When he turned it, it was smooth, more like a tuning knob on a radio. But as he turned it, the Hutu/Tutsi atrocities on the set fuzzed out to be replaced by another crystal clear image.

The next program appeared to be a World War II movie: Japanese infantry troops moving down a crude city street, kicking down doors, firing at civilians as they fled, tossing grenades into windows. Buildings were set ablaze, yet from some, soldiers dragged screaming Asian women out into the street, beat them senseless, and proceeded to rape them. Some soldiers took turns with the women, but when the rapes were concluded, the soldiers sliced off each woman's breasts and tossed them aside. Vulvas and clitorises were cut off, and bayonets sunk deep into vaginas and rectums. Then the soldiers walked away, leaving the women to cringe in the dirt and the town to burn behind them.

Farthing collapsed to his knees, quite close to being sick to his stomach for the second time tonight. But in the process, his finger had nudged the channel knob the slightest bit. The screen fuzzed out, then refocused onto some kind of a conveyor platform. On either side of the platform stood a man, each wearing a yellow rubberized rain suit with a hood and plastic face shield. The conveyor was moving, and eventually there came something into view: a spread-legged nude woman with long blond hair. She was unconscious, but then one of the men roused her by emptying a glass of water in her face. Each man grabbed an ankle and hauled her forward just as she was coming to. What Farthing didn't notice until now was the massive band saw at the end of the platform; the woman barely had time to realize her end before she was briskly dragged through the band saw, which bisected her from crotch to head. Her two halves flopped off the table.

She had to have been eight-months pregnant.

Then one of the men nonchalantly hosed off the platform, and that's when Farthing passed out.

More aggravating than the bell at a fire station was the sound Farthing awoke to; it was loud, obnoxious, and terrifying, and did nothing but exacerbate the ache throbbing in his skull thanks to last night's excess of alcohol. Eventually, he sat up, finding himself mysteriously relocated into his late-uncle's big four-poster bed. The last thing he remembered was collapsing to his knees last night before that old television in the back room.

How did I get here? he wondered. Must've crawled … and then he winced again when that "fire-bell" sounded once more. "Fuck …" Of course, it was the phone, not a cellphone but the kind that needed to be plugged into a phone line. *My first phone call as an Englander,* he thought.

Just before it would ring a third time, he snatched it up and said in a rather gravelly voice, "Uh, hello?"

There was a hollow pause, then a British-accented voice replied, "Have you found it yet?"

Was this a telemarketer? "Found what? Who is this?"

"Did he leave anything … Instructions, perhaps?"

"Who the fuck is this?" Farthing demanded in his loudest Ugly American voice.

click.

"Fuckers." He ground his teeth at the blade of harsh sunlight cutting through the gap in the drapes. *What was I doing last night?* he asked himself, but then, *Oh, shit, that's right. I was watching that old television, and—*

Recollection truncated the rest of the thought. The TV set had been working, and on it he'd seen the most abominable broadcast. When he strained his fogged memory, he gulped, dredging up specific images of horror that he could never have imagined: murders, mutilations—it all made his head spin now. His sentience felt as skewed as a pile of fruit in a blender. Children being swallowed whole by pythons before a cheering crowd, prisoners being fed roasted human arms, and the grand finale, the pregnant woman being perfunctorily halved by a band saw.

The urge to vomit crept up, but he managed to quell it in time. He'd thrown up in the yard last night, hadn't he? That acrid after-taste remained in his mouth. Still partly dizzy, he stumbled to the bathroom, took a shower, then brushed his teeth and gargled for five minutes. Thank God Uncle Eldred's mouth wash remained.

It must've been some internet shit I saw last night, he considered. *The Dark Net, the Dark Web,* whatever they were calling it. These days it was impossible not to hear of such realities. Untraceable purveyors of child pornography, genuine rapes, snuff films, and the like. How much of this Farthing actually believed, he was in no position to say, but all told, after what he'd seen last night?

He navigated himself to the back room, hesitantly approached the TV set, and turned it on. Of course, nothing happened. How could it? There was no power source and not even a plug to connect to an outlet.

Then the simplest conclusion occurred to him.

I must've dreamed it. I dreamed all that shit, and

the vision in the backyard too, the two guys digging up the grave. This was easier to accept … or at least it was for a moment. Dreaming all those horrific images meant that it all came from *him,* from his own subconscious. *My own mind manufactured that sick shit.* A morbid man he was not, and hoped he was not becoming, so why would his dreaming mind stage such a display of abhorrence?

"Just one of those things," he muttered. "Combination of too much alcohol, jet lag, and the hub-bub of moving to a new place … But mostly alcohol."

That conclusion would do for now. It was noon already, the day half-wasted, and he was determined to make a better start to his resettlement here. There was much to do, and he'd first have to discern what steps needed be taken to legally establish residence. He'd need to apply for new credit cards.

He nearly swore aloud when the phone rang again. Fuming, he picked up the extension in the room.

"Yes?"

It was not a British accent that replied this time but something more difficult to identify. Something sharper, edgier. Eastern European, maybe? "Um, yes. I would like to know if—if you

94

have any questions."

"WHO THE FUCK IS THIS?" Farthing blared.

"Oh, I see, yes. I guess no one has talked to you …"

"Talked to me about what?"

They hung up.

What IS this shit? What kind of telemarketers are these?

Farthing, as it has probably been observed by now, was a bit of a grouch, a "grumpy old man." New things and new ways he did not respond well to, and the raging hangover only compounded these inconveniences. *If just one more of these rude motherfuckers calls, why, I'll …* But of course, he didn't really know *what he'd do except answer the phone.*

He looked down again at the dead television. "Fucker," he said. Some several feet in front of the set, though, he noticed four indentations in the carpet, as if his uncle had placed a chair precisely in the same spot. Then he remembered the fold-down metal chair leaning against the back wall. He couldn't resist …

He took up the chair, opened it, and, as he'd pretty much predicted, found that the four rubber-capped ends of the chair legs fit perfectly into the four carpet indentations.

So Uncle Eldred was definitely watching this TV, he thought, drawing the logical conclusion. Watching a TV with no power cord. By himself. In the biggest room in the house but one that has nothing else in it.

He put the chair back; his head ached too severely to think too hard on the matter. Food was more paramount than these stray ruminations, but he still was unaware of any food that might have remained in the trailer after his uncle's passing. He was about to turn out of the room and proceed to the kitchen, but then his eye snagged on something, for whatever reason. It was the wheeled wooden stand on which the old television sat. Several drawers had been mounted near the top.

Farthing bent over and opened one.

What the shit is this?

He recognized what the drawer contained: blood transfusion bags. They were unopened and wrapped in clear plastic. A front label read K-SHIELD ADVANTAGE BLOOD DRAW KIT - STERILE WHEN UNOPENED.

This suggested some things, didn't it? It made sense that a man his uncle's age might have health problems. Perhaps one of them was a blood disorder.

Hmm.

Some other plastic bags in the same drawer

contained plastic tubing and packets of blood-draw needles. *He must've had a home-care nurse come here sometimes, to draw blood for analysis?* Farthing wondered. *Maybe he was on dialysis. Don't they have home-dialysis now?*

His stomach growled, compelling him to make a fast-track to the kitchen. The refrigerator contained only beer and some condiments. He flapped open and closed the upper kitchen cabinets, finding most empty. One, however, contained Morrison's Cornflakes. He opened the box and inner bag, and stuffed several handfuls rapidly into his mouth. *Just like Kellogg's!* he assessed. It was with some eagerness that he opened the next cupboard, hoping for something of a treat.

Instead, his mouth fell open and his eyes crossed. The cupboard contained multiple cans of something with the label: SPOTTED DICK.

"What the fuck!"

He almost yelled next when someone began knocking on the front door, quite loudly, and at the same time, the phone rang again.

"For shit's sake!" and he answered the phone: "Hello!"

Another accented voice, Middle Eastern, perhaps. "Oh, hello. Eeze Eeldred there pleeze?"

"No, he's dead!"

"Oh, I see. And who might theese be?"

"Theese is the person who leeves here now and is about to hang the fuck up on you!" Farthing yelled, and hung up. His shoulders hunched when the door knocker resounded, louder now. *This is too much!* He rushed to the door, yanked it open, was about to yell but—

"Ah, Mr. Farthing," greeted Cooper with his usual big bearded smile. "I do hope my unannounced visit has not in any way presented a disruption to your day."

Farthing at once calmed down; in fact, he was happy to see Cooper. "No disruption at all. Please come in."

Cooper nodded and entered, but seemed to cast a strange eye to his host. "I do hope your first night in Burnstow was a pleasant one, but—if I may say it—you don't seem all the fresher for your night's rest."

"That's quite true, Mr. Cooper. And if I appear hungover, it's because, well, I'm hungover."

"Ah, yes, sir. The blessing of alcohol and also its accommodating malediction. But I've stopped round to ask a question or two—"

"And I've got a question for *you*, Mr. Cooper," and he almost testily made his way back to the kitchen cupboard. "Like what the hell is Spotted

Dick?" and he held up one of the cans.

Cooper's abdomen ballooned forth when he leaned back and laughed. "I can easily understand why such a title would seem strange to American eyes. But spotted dick is simply a delightful British dessert, a bit akin to bread pudding, I should think."

This surprised Farthing but … *With a name like that, I can't POSSIBLY eat it.*

"I'm sure you'll acclimate quite well to our British cuisine," added Cooper, "and all else as well. But I've come to just remind you that there are several matters that will soon need your attention. As I am not only the executor of your uncle's will, I was also, as I've made you aware, a personal friend. It would be helpful for you to visit my office in the near future, in order that you might sign the final probate termination, the title deed, some insurance odds and ends, if you'd like to continue with them. And any other matters that may come to your mind, all my pleasure to take care of for you free of charge." The portly man laughed again. "You see, not *all lawyers are intent on squeezing blood out of rocks.*"

What a nice guy. "That's very generous of you, Mr. Cooper, and I will indeed come by your office soon." But the remark about *blood out of rocks instantly refreshed Farthing's curiosity. "Do you happen to know if my uncle had any blood diseases, or ailments that might require transfusions?"*

Cooper straightened his posture at once. "I am pretty certain, sir, that I am aware of no such thing. He did not, in fact, keep me apprised, in any form, shape, or way, of his medical disposition."

"Hmm, yes. So I guess his cause of death can pretty much be summed up to old age?"

Cooper nodded grimly. "Myocardial infarction, according to his death certificate. I'll pass it on to you as well as all other pertinent paperwork when you come by. And any transfers of banking information, reciprocities, and whatnot, I'm all too happy to take care of."

"Thank you."

"And what plans do you have in mind for today?"

Farthing sighed. "Probably a nap until the hangover goes away. Up till now, I've been receiving a bunch of annoying phone calls—telemarketers, I guess, but so far, it's not clear what they're selling."

"The bane of all good folk, I'm afraid—telemarketers. There's no getting around them, I'm sorry to say. They should be pilloried, the lot of them."

"Oh, and that weird television in the back room," Farthing thought to add. "I don't remember what you said about it yesterday, but … did you ever happen to see it turned on?"

Cooper pulled up, eyeing Farthing most directly. "In the lengths of my powers of recollection, Mr. Farthing, I am left to respond to your question in a negative mode—what I mean is, in a very dearth of verbiage, no, I never once saw the television on or in any manner of use. Additionally, as we both observed yesterday, since the set appears to possess no power cord, I can only suppose that the cord was accidentally yanked out."

Sometimes, listening to Cooper answer a simple question left Farthing winded. "Well, doesn't that strike you as strange?"

Cooper seemed to ruminate upon the question and appeared to be about to commence with something of a disquisition. "Well, sir, I'm afraid I am utterly unequipped to give answer to your question, considering, of course, the very subjective nature of the word *strange.* Who am I, after all, to make such a judgment about another man's conceptions? I might select a different word to reflect your meaning, such as *peculiar* or *extraordinary, in which case I would have to assent, yes. Keeping a television that doesn't operate might seem peculiar to most."*

Farthing's thoughts stalled. *A television that doesn't operate ...* But last night, it *did seem to operate, did it not? But—No, no, no! he ordered himself. That was all a nightmare. I'm sure it was!* "Can you shed any light on why Uncle Eldred might've kept that back room the way he did?"

Cooper stroked his beard very briefly. "Let's look, shall we? Since I'm not quite grasping your meaning," and then both men went down the hall.

In the room so indicated, Farthing went on, "See? Isn't it strange—er, I should say peculiar— that my uncle reserved the largest bedroom in the trailer to house little more than this clunker TV? And you can see right here"—Farthing pointed down to the four indentations in the carpet, then pointed to the chair on the back wall—"my uncle obviously used to place that chair in this spot, right in front of the set. Why would he sit in front of a non-working television, in a room *this large, all by himself?"*

"You've duped me yet again, sir!" Copper allowed in his usual high spirits. "It would demand a keener intelligence than my own, I'm afraid, to make any fitting response to what you ask—except other than this—and, mind, I wouldn't suggest such a possibility if you hadn't pressed me. What

I mean is ... Let me resort to the infuriating tactic of answering a question with a question, so not to seem blunt." Cooper raised a finger, as if about to dispense a significant wisdom. "Would it be, say, reasonable, for one to advance the possibility, or even—dear me—the likelihood, that a man of your uncle's very many years, in the deepest twilight of his life among us, that he was, er, or might be—"

Farthing rolled his eyes. "Of course! That he'd gone crazy. I'd say that's a *very* reasonable theory to suggest, and since you knew him so well, do you think that that was the case? That Uncle Eldred had grown mentally deficient, senile, or just plain nuts?"

Cooper reflected the words, then nodded curtly. "No, Mr. Farthing. In my *personal* observation, not the least trace of mental illness or any manner of cognitive impairment did he ever exhibit in my presence, nor did I ever overhear such a thing from anyone else. But one can never know, can they?"

"Yeah, you're right." Farthing was looking down at the floor. "Plenty of people go nuts, and no one ever even notices. It makes me feel like a schmuck now."

"Really, sir, a schmuck? I think you're taking too blistering a view on the matter."

"Maybe," Farthing added. "I should've made

103

better efforts to contact him. I should've visited him. He left me this place and a bunch of money, he left me set for life, and I never even bothered to come and see him."

Cooper consolingly patted Farthing's shoulder. "You can take it from me, sir, when I say that your uncle was not despondent in the least, nor lonely, nor dejected. I can honestly say that I never saw him with anything less than a smile on his face."

Well, that's good, at least. It was a strange recognition, though. His uncle had died alone in this very trailer. One day, more than likely, so would Farthing.

"Ah," Cooper piped up again, "I see now what spurred your question about ailments of the blood." The drawer in the TV stand remained open, plainly showing the unopened blood bags. "Yet another mystery that I'm afraid I'm of no use in solving."

Farthing was about to ask if Cooper knew of any other women who'd posed for Eldred, but—

"Not again!"

—the phone rang.

"Excuse me," then Farthing snapped up the phone. "Hello?"

Dead air for a moment, then, "Have you been having the dreams yet?"

"What dreams?" Farthing barked. "Who the fuck is this?"

"Mind your dreams." Then, *click.*

This time, the caller's accent had sounded French, and female, perhaps.

"More telemarketers, I take it?" Cooper asked.

"If they are, they suck. They're not telling me what they're selling. They might be people who knew my uncle but don't know he's dead."

"Hmm," Cooper remarked. "Another mystery, I dare say. Did I hear you say something about dreams?"

"Yeah, the asshole on the phone asked me if I'd been having dreams." Farthing frowned. "What kind of thing is *that* for someone to ask?"

"I can't imagine ..." The interruptions were causing conversation to stagnate, so Cooper continued, "Now I'm afraid I must scurry back to the office, for more of the burdens of employment are beckoning. Come in at your leisure to sign those papers, if you will." Cooper clicked his heels and bowed. "And now I bid you a wonderful day."

"Thanks. Later." Farthing doubted that the word *wonderful* would apply to any aspect of him until the headache was gone. More food seemed in order, something more substantial than corn flakes and, no ... spotted dick would *not* be on today's menu.

A sun-shiny day greeted him when he left the trailer, which improved his mood, yet the glare of the sun cut into his headache like a blade. He exited the quiet park, making a few cursory nods to distant residents walking their dogs or retrieving mail. It was just across Main Street where he found the wooden ramp to the beach.

That's more like it, he thought.

This wasn't peak season, but there were still a few vacationers walking the beach and bobbing out in the surf. And it wasn't baking hot here either. *Must be low tide,* he figured; there were several hundred yards of beach extending outward. Halfway down, however, an old brick foundation stuck out of the sand, probably a hotel finally torn down ahead of the corroding beach. *Good ole Global Warming ...* Old anchors and capstans remained half-buried, and closer in, he could see the long black groins of larch and oak set in place in an attempt to forestall further beach erosion. He wondered how many more decades it would take for the tide to reach Main Street. *Hopefully, I'll be dead by then ...*

He shielded his eyes and gazed west: there was only endless beach, dunes, and a wall of slightly bent trees. Of people, there were none—

No! A lone figure could be seen far off when

Farthing squinted. The figure seemed to be walking at a sturdy pace, but after a few minutes, Farthing looked again and the figure seemed to have exhibited no progress. Obviously, an illusion of the distance and the visual monotony of the vast stretch of sand.

Then he turned and looked east. This might be more promising. First, set out in ranks were rows and rows of wooden beach chairs and umbrellas. Beyond, he spotted myriad salt-box-style beach houses and some impressive waterfront homes. Yet before that there stretched an inviting length of boardwalk, complete with tourist gift shops and eateries, a bumper-car arena, and a modest Ferris wheel.

His aging legs trudged toward this location, for delectable smells enticed him from wheeled vendors' carts. Once on the boardwalk, a typical snide Brit voice heckled him. "Ah, just what we need—another bloomin' American!"

Farthing looked first at the steaming cart, over which hung a side that read BANGERS - PIPING HOT!, and then at the proprietor, a long-necked, clean-shaven character wearing one of those shifty newsboy hats. He looked about Farthing's age.

"How could you tell I'm American?"

"Easy, you clothes don't fit proper, and you

do look like a bloke nursin' a bad hangover. You Yanks, can't handle a pint—"

Jeez, it shows that easily?

"—but for that, I'd advise ya try our tried-and-true cure—a couple 'a bangers."

Farthing stared. "What's a banger?"

The proprietor smiled. "Know what a fuckin' hot dog is, sir?"

"Yeah, I think so."

"Same thing, mate."

"Okay, I'll take two."

"Right-o!"

Two Oscar Meyer hot dogs on rolls were passed to Farthing, who wolfed one down quickly. Then the proprietor, who was leaning over the cart on his elbows, said, "Bet you're wonderin' where the beach whores is, eh?"

The thought, of course, did not occur to Farthing, but he saw no harm in answering, "Yeah, where?"

The Brit slapped his hand down hard on the top of the cart. "There ain't any!" and then he burst into a roar of laughter.

Must be my aura ...

The proprietor pointed across the way, to an open bar made of wooden slats. The sign read THE WET YOUR WHISTLE PUB. Mostly men, older than Farthing, sat inside, stolid-faced over mugs of beer.

"But long back, there use ta be a barmaid there, Debbie she was called. Had one tit bigger than the other, I swear, and when you had 'em both in your face the same time, it were like havin' two girls at once, it was! And she'd work the beer taps with one hand and work your cock with the other, all for like five pounds. More 'n' a little 'a *my* jism on the floor over there, I can tell ya," he laughed. "Oh, and the pub in town, place called Mattshaw's. They got a hefty tit-wagon over there named Bernice—"

Farthing's brow instantly popped up.

"—as nice a bird as you could ever meet on a May mornin'. But what I hear is if ya go there just afore closin' time and got some righteous coin in yer pocket, she'd be more 'n' happy to let you top off her gravy boat." The man pointed. "Ah, and have an eyeball on *these* two sausage jockeys."

Farthing looked up and saw two young but shapely and very endowed girls in bright bikinis walking by, yakking in heavy English accents. They were attractive, yes, but—

"Come on, man," Farthing chastised. "Those girls look fifteen."

The hot dog man shook his head. "You know like that say. If there's grass on the field … you play ball!" And then came another roar of laughter.

This guy's killing me, Farthing thought, but before he could separate himself from this situation, the guy asked, "Here on holiday, are ya?"

"No, actually, I inherited a property nearby, and I've decided to live here."

"Good for you, mate. Where ya live?"

Farthing pointed across the street. "The trailer park over there."

"Oh, you live at the Magnus, do ya? Nice park." The proprietor nodded; something about that newsboy hat made him look disreputable and dishonest. "But 'twas a funny thing I 'eard about it back in the day—jolly odd, actually."

This tweaked Farthing's interest. "What funny thing?"

The proprietor's eyes thinned, as one drifting into reminiscence. "I knew a bird—shit, mate, probably back when John Major was PM. Now, I was a young bloke back then and could lay pipe with the best of 'em—"

Lay pipe, Farthing thought. *Just what I need to hear about.*

"—and I had me my share 'a women, but there was this one gal, Carla, her name was, and she were a looker, I'll tell ya that much … from the neck down is what I mean. 'Ad a body on her like Diana Rigg in that shitty Bond flick and a face like, well, maybe like Peter Cushing …"

The image projected into Farthing's mind gave him a jolt.

"But who looks at the face anyway, eh? And I don't wanna say she was a whore, but, well, fuck it—she was a whore. And she could do that tongue thing, ya know, what like some gals can do? Be suckin' yer John Thomas and lickin' yer arsehole the same time? Ya know?"

"Ah, no," Farthing admitted.

"I guess she were what Yanks would call a *cum dumpster, yeah?*"

This time, Farthing almost choked on the last of his hot dog.

"And there I was, proud as can be, walkin' down the street holdin' her hand and playin' kissy face with her and not even *thinkin' that* them same lips I'm kissin' have been wrapped around damn near every cock in Sussex, but, fuck it, ya know? Anyway, ya know what she tell me, this Carla? What she tell me about Magnus Park?"

Farthing didn't think he wanted to know, but he could not forswear asking. "Uh, what?"

"She tell me there were a older bloke livin' there, a feller with full pockets, who she'd 'eard were kind of a kink —"

Farthing's eyes got wider. "Yeah?"

"But he didn't try nothin' on with her, nothin' kinky or sexual, I mean. But he offer her two hunnert pounds fer—blimey, it been *years* since't I even *thought 'a* this—but he pay her two hunnert pounds to—and what ya gotta understand, mate, is back then two hunnert pounds were worth a *lot* more 'n' it is today—"

Farthing was wearing out.

"Anyway, he pay her all that money for a pint of her blood."

Farthing stared. Silence fell like a wall.

An older guy, kinky, with money? At the same trailer park? Farthing couldn't help but reason the person to which the hot dog guy referred was probably Uncle Eldred.

He waited for a punch line. "What? Let me guess. He was a vampire?"

"No, no, mate, how could he be? This were broad daylight, she tell me, and everything I ever heerd 'bout vampires say they can't be in daylight."

"So why the hell did this guy pay your girlfriend for a pint of her blood?" Farthing demanded, getting a bit irked. "If he needed a transfusion, he could just go to the hospital and get it, right? For free? You have nationalized healthcare, don't you?"

"That we do, mate, unlike some *less sophisticated*

countries out there, but that we do."

"Well, what did Carla say? She must've asked the guy why he wanted her blood."

The proprietor shrugged. "Can't say as I recall, and I weren't much thinkin' on it. What ya gotta understand about Carla, see, she had a way of takin' a fella's thoughts off 'a anything but what's ridin' uptown—"

Farthing smirked. "Uptown?"

"That's how good her tits was. A regular apple-dumpling cart."

"Well, didn't you ask her? She must've inquired. How could she not? If someone wanted to buy *my blood, I'd sure as hell ask them why."*

"Look, mate, sure, I guess it struck me as odd, but all's I was doin' was workin' 'er up for a piece of arse."

But the coincidence was too much to let go. Not just the reference to a kinky older guy in the same park but then Farthing had also found those blood-collection bags in the trailer. *This is too fuckin' much.* "What about—wait!" he started. "Does Carla still live around here? I'd love to ask her about it myself."

"No chance, mate," said the proprietor. "Carla split not long after. Was everyone's question for the better part of a year, where she went, I mean.

She had herself lots of friends, but she didn't leave none of 'em—nor yet myself— forwarding address. Not even so much as a peep beforehand that she were leavin' town." He stirred the pot of hot dogs. "Be damned if anyone ever heerd from her again."

Farthing bought two more hot dogs, and to the shifty proprietor, he bid as pleasant a farewell as he could muster. Two more hot dogs would just be the ticket, he thought, to relieve the hangover. He went back out to the beach to eat, watch the incoming tide, and espy whatever girls in bikinis might wander into his field of vision. A glance left showed him that same distant beach-walker he'd seen when he arrived, who appeared still to be walking but did not seem to be making any progress. It looked more like a chess piece. Last night, he'd dreamed that he'd mistaken a black post for a black-clad person. And speaking of dreams …

The commotion of the last two days, not to mention the time change, had left Farthing overcome by sudden exhaustion, and he dozed off right there on the beach bench, the regularity of the surf-sounds lulling him pleasantly.

But no pleasantness followed him from this moment on.

It must be a dream, yes, but it seemed to unfold from a different perspective, as dreams sometimes did. This time, the dream was straight-on first-person, but he received the distinct notion that he *wasn't* seeing the dream's entails through his own eyes. His perspective seemed to be hovering in a way, and passing through solid objects, like cars on a street and even through the walls of some sort of one-story office building, a doctor's office, it looked like, or a clinic.

Farthing's awareness passed through the front double glass doors, then another wall. Now he could see a front office and an Asian woman in business attire sitting at a desk.

Then, through the next wall he went, into not another office but some kind of a medical suite. There was little time to assess what was taking place. Another Asian woman, hugely pregnant and dressed in a hospital gown, lay on an exam table, unconscious by the look of the IV line going into her arm. Her bare ankles were hooked into metal stirrups, which widely opened her legs.

It couldn't be more clear what was occurring: a late-term abortion.

A face-masked doctor sat on a stool between

the patient's legs; a similarly masked nurse stood aside.

The patient's pubic area was completely divested of hair, and in the obvious opening between her legs, a bald baby's head was visible. The head was moving.

The nurse passed the doctor a large syringe with a heavy-gauge needle, and the doctor unhesitantly jammed the needle tip into the crown of the baby's skull. Even a tiny *crunch was heard. The nurse looked away. The doctor depressed the syringe's plunger and emptied its contents into the fetus's* brain.

The head then stopped moving.

The doctor grabbed the fetus's throat and, with one long pull, evacuated the baby from the patient's womb. There was an indescribable wet sound that accompanied this process.

The umbilicus was snipped. The dead baby was then placed in a shiny metal trough, in which it lay motionless. The doctor said something in an Asian language, and then the nurse made an undecipherable reply. Her arms moved in some precision as she reeled out the remainder of the umbilicus and also the entire placenta from the patient's agape vaginal aperture. This meaty debris was all dropped into another shiny metal pan.

But when the nurse turned, her eyes shot wide

over her mask, she pointed and gasped some exclamation in her native language. The doctor swiveled on his stool, took a visual note of the problem, and uttered some manner of curse.

The aborted baby on the table was still moving.

The doctor stood up, lurching into action. A mechanical revving sound rose as he hoisted up a high-powered oscillating orthopedic bone saw and expertly separated the full-grown fetus's head from its body. It wobbled around a little on the table, then stopped, bright fresh blood dribbling from the neck.

Farthing, in the dream, felt like he was suffocating and falling in a spiral. He could've been a bullet spinning out of its barrel. There came an impression that he was soaring through space, or time, or both. He could not understand. Was there a chuckling behind this dreamscape in his mind? It seemed so.

Next thing he saw, high in a desert sunset, was an immense Bauhausian palace with great pillars and slabs of polished granite. Many vehicles, including military vehicles, were parked in ranks in the palace's front. Many soldiers stood guard at various openings; they were *not adorned in US uniforms, nor did any familiar flags fly before the palace. Instead*, it was a flag of one red stripe, one white, and one black. Farthing didn't have a clue …

But his dreaming point of view flew up the high hill, passed more soldiers at attention, and then bored through stone walls, as had been his experience at the atrocious clinic. Interior fountains burbled, stone walls shined like glass. It was a sedate, quiet vision until—

Farthing, even in the dream or whatever it was, flinched severely at the long, grinding sound of a female scream. Now his perspective slid through more interior stone walls. Several rooms seemed to be vaults guarded by more perfectly still soldiers, while in the middle of each vault there stood wooden pallets on which were stacked veritable piles of banded US currency. These piles stood man-tall.

Farthing realized, *That has to be hundreds of millions of US dollars just sitting there …*

But the screaming grew louder and more horrifying as he soared onward. In one small room, he saw gruff soldiers primitively drowning a shirtless man in a bucket of water, but as Farthing's perspective edged closer, he could first *smell* and then *see* that it was not water but diarrhea. The soldiers held the victim down for a long time, laughing as the final twitches ceased and the last of the man's breath bubbled up out of the brown, lumpy broth. If Farthing had had a stomach in the dream, it surely would've emptied just then.

Next, some unknown force shoved him through another wall, this time into a room—

No no no! I can't see this!

—where soldiers were perfunctorily raping naked children on long tables, quite like autopsy tables. Some children were crying and shuddering in shock, while others just lay there with staring eyes and opened mouths.

Out! Out! Farthing screamed at himself, and, thank God, his sentience obeyed; his horror shot him through another thick stone wall.

But relief was short-lived. The next room proved to be the very source of the insane female screams he'd heard previously.

He took one look, again ordered himself *Out! Out!* but this time didn't budge.

He just hung there, like vapor, in mid-air while something he couldn't understand forced him to watch …

A nude, dark-haired woman lay outstretched on the stone floor, wrists and ankles splayed by shackles. Several soldiers looked down, smiling, some with bulges at their crotches. But one soldier knelt beside the woman, and he—

SNIP! SNIP! SNIP!

—cut off her nose with something like tin-shears, then both of her ears. Most of her fingers and toes had already been clipped off. The kneeling soldier nodded, then pulled out each nipple with forefinger and thumb, and—

SNIP! SNIP!

The woman's throat emitted screams more like jammed gears in a machine. She shuddered, jerking against her shackles with repeated mad *clacking* sounds, her back arched, the whites of her eyes now fully red.

Next, the soldier looked up, jabbered something in his native language, and then the other soldiers parted. One came back with nothing more terrifying than a green rubber garden hose. But then two more soldiers, both wearing heavy asbestos gloves, walked awkwardly into view, each bearing the handle of a steaming steel pot. Farthing was able to look *into* the pot, and what he saw was something like molten green plastic, slowly bubbling. The pot must've held ten gallons, twenty, perhaps. Farthing could even smell that unmistakable stench of melted plastic. There was no dramatic prelude. The two soldiers, without further pause, emptied the pot's steaming contents onto the woman, coating her from neck to groin. There was no point in describing her shrieks nor her physical convulsions as the bubbling plastic fizzed into her most sensitive skin. The pot was moved away; the kneeling solider rose and stepped back, then nodded to the soldier with the hose.

Great billows of steam mushroomed up when the one soldier opened the hose valve and inundated the plastic on the woman with cold water. This process continued for a few minutes, until it was sure that the hot plastic was now sufficiently cooled and hardened.

The woman, somehow, was still alive, her eyes crazy and her mouth opening and closing but no longer proffering screams.

Another order was barked, then four soldiers leaned over, hooked their fingers underneath the shell of hardened plastic, then yanked that shell right off, along with the woman's skin. The sound of that almost cost Farthing his consciousness …

At once, however, the tone of mind-warping atrocity was punctured by the simple sound of one person slowly clapping his hands.

It was a man walking across the room, having just witnessed the torture. Farthing recognized the man: the long-dead Saddam Hussein.

Farthing awoke winded, like someone who'd

just barely escaped killers. He jerked upright on the beach bench and felt more alarmed when he realized it was nighttime and the tide had crawled almost up to the boardwalk. *Damn it to Hell,* he groaned to himself, rising from the bench. He wobbled a moment. *I ate hot dogs from that guy, then fell asleep and had the worst dreams of my life. Welcome to fuckin' England.*

Behind him now, the boardwalk was lit up; arcade bells were ringing. People were playing games like ring toss, water-gun rifle range, bumper cars, and the like. Farthing noticed the Ferris wheel was revolving and alit. Various folks milled about, laughing, snacking, having fun, but Farthing felt, instead, grim.

The blinking lights at the WET YOUR WHISTLE PUB seemed to seduce him—a cold beer would go nicely right now—but he willed himself away and back down the beach; he'd learned long ago that the theorem of Hair of the Dog was a myth.

He felt harassed by snippets of his atrocious dreams; his shoulders hunched as he walked as if he at any moment expected to be pounced upon by an unknown entity. Farther down the beach and away from the gaily lit boardwalk, he felt paranoid, he felt watched; in fact, he kept straining his vision forward, wondering if that lone walker he'd seen earlier was still there, but it was too dark to tell and, in fact, ridiculous to ponder such a thing. Moonlight glimmered on the sea to his left, and nothing more.

Finally, he cut across off the beach and made his way back to the trailer park, which looked different now; it looked smaller, the units appeared closer together. This was strange because things usually looked larger in darkness than light. A lump in a barely lit window could've been a head; a swoosh above him gave him a start; it must have been an unseen night bird. He heard a large dog barking but couldn't guess from which direction it came.

Fourth Street finally found him; he turned and walked faster down the dark street. It seemed odd that absolutely no one was about, not even a single dog-walker. At the end of the street, where his uncle's trailer was, a dark car idled by very slowly; it had the look of an expensive sports car. *These assholes again!* he thought, but he was too tired to run after the vehicle. From the opposite direction, however, that is, just behind him, a weathered woman's voice said, "Eldred? My word! Is that you?"

Farthing spun around, wincing into misaligned headlights. It was an old red car that rumbled up behind him. He waited for it to stop and looked into the open driver's window, but before he could see anything, he nearly gagged. *Oh, God!*

A deep stench of urine eddied from the window, right into Farthing's frowning face, and at once, he thought, *Finally. The Piss Car Lady …*

"N-no, I'm not Eldred. He was my uncle, and I'm afraid he died recently …"

Only wedges of the woman were visible in the dicey park light: old white straggly hair up in a bun, a thin but jowly face, very thick glasses. "Oh, I didn't know," she said in a standard old-lady voice. "Lord have mercy … not that I expect he had much use for the Lord," and then she cracked an unpleasant laugh.

"What? Why do you say that?"

She either didn't hear his question or was choosing to ignore it. "I'm Eloise. Eldred's been me friend for a very long time. I'm so sorry he's passed on. He used to help me on occasion …"

Farthing remembered Cooper saying something similar, about Eldred's generosity to panhandlers and the like. But it was hard for him to focus on this woman, this Eloise, due to the revolting stench wafting out of the car. She seemed to be wearing a threadbare manner of summer dress with some holes in the shoulders; her thin face was ashen-gray, and her eyes sunken deep into their sockets:

124

nearly a living skull.

"I was so hopin' against all hope I'd find Eldred—" The sunken blood-shot eyes opened wide and appraised him. "Why, you look so much like him! But anyway, I thought he might be worryin' about me because I hadn't been by for so long. See, I was … away for a while."

"Oh, vacation?" Farthing pressed. He was curious to know; Cooper had suspected she was dead.

"No. I'm afraid I was in the hospital, young man—"

The remark amused Farthing, for he was anything but a *young man. But Eloise, by the looks of her, must be in her late-eighties.*

"—but I'm fine now, just fine, by the grace of God. I'm hoping you might be able to help an old woman out. Like your uncle used to."

"I'm sorry, Eloise, but I don't have any cash on me. You see, I just moved to Burnstow yesterday."

"Oh, how lovely." She seemed worse than disappointed but trying to conceal that. "Moving into your uncle's old place, are you?"

"That's right."

The old woman paused. "Are you—er. Might you be … taking up with that bunch of his?"

Farthing looked crookedly at her. "That

125

bunch? What bunch is that?"

"Them ritzos is what I mean," she grated. "Did your uncle ever have a word with you about them or that business they was up to?"

Suddenly, this was getting so interesting, he could tolerate the piss-stench. "Eloise, are you talking about the people who've been driving by here in very expensive cars?"

"Don't you trust 'em, not that bunch. Richer than King Croesus, the lot of 'em." Now her thoughts seemed to sidetrack her into some bitter recollection. "But do ya think they'd ever help *me out*—no, I don't think so. Oh, they were all about it when I was givin' 'em what Eldred needed, but when they was done with me—blast the lot of 'em. And then there was that one bitch—a foreigner, she was, from some God forsaken place. She'd laugh at me and tell me in *her country,* people'd be worked to death. People like me weren't worth nothin' to no one."

This was getting unpleasant as well as sad. Farthing noted tears in the old woman's eyes. *What the hell is she talking about? The people in the fancy cars?* "Eloise," he began, fishing around in his pockets. He did indeed have some stray bills there. "I was wrong. I *do* have a little bit of money on me. Here, you can have it."

He passed her the crumpled bills, and her ancient eyes lit up. "Oh, bless you, young man. I ain't got much petrol left, and I ain't eaten much of anything since they let me out. Bless you."

He leaned in closer. "But what did you mean when you said you'd given them what Eldred needed?"

When she answered, Farthing saw that she had no teeth. "Swore I'd never say," she whispered, "but I guess it don't matter a rip now since Eldred's in the grave …"

"No, Eloise, I'm sure it doesn't. So what was it? What was it he needed?"

She held up a withered, liver-spotted arm; loose skin hung off the bone like a flag. "See those? See those there?" She was pointing to what Farthing assumed were liver-spots. "That's what he needed, him 'n' that lot. They needed blood. So I sold 'em mine any chance I got, 'cos by then I wasn't the looker I'd been back in the day, and I needed money just like anyone."

They weren't liver spots; they were old needle marks.

You've gotta be shitting me, Farthing thought in shock. *Blood. These people bought BLOOD from her. Just like the hot dog guy's girlfriend!*

"So, Eloise," he began carefully. "You mean

these rich people … they *paid* you to give your blood to them?"

"That they did. Even had a nurse there with 'em, to put the needle in proper," Eloise revealed. "'Least, they *said she were a nurse.*"

Farthing felt mind-boggled, staring at this old woman.

"Every two, three months as I recall. That nurse girl said it weren't safe to take no more 'n that. But I don't think they gave a blast. They could'a bled me dry right there and wouldn't've cared one way or other. But it weren't just me they used; it were a bunch 'a girls, you know, whores on the drugs, vagrants, folks like what'd do *anything* for money."

Now Farthing's curiosity was ticking like a clock. He leaned closer to the old woman. "Eloise. Please. Tell me. Tell me why my Uncle Eldred needed your blood."

She looked at him; her face appeared dead. "In cahoots, they all was—with Eldred, I mean. That's why he were so rich—that bunch, they gave him money because, because 'a what Eldred could do. See, Eldred had … talents, I guess you could call it. He could show 'em things they wanted ta see," and then she broke off and began coughing. Suddenly, she was hitching where she sat, wheezing like an asthmatic.

My God, lady! Don't die! "Eldred showed them things? Who? Who did he show? The rich people with the fancy cars?"

Eloise hacked a few more times, nodding.

"What things did Eldred show them?" he pleaded. "I don't understand. And what does it have to do with them paying you for your blood?"

The lady coughed once more, ferociously. "Don't get involved with them awful folks, trust me. I got to get to the BP right away, son, afore I run outta petrol. But hear me well. Don't get involved with any 'a that mess. And stay away from that goddamned telly," and with that, she coughed again, spat out what appeared to be bloody phlegm, and drove off.

Farthing stared after her. He could still hear her coughing as she got to the park exit.

The goddamned TELLY? Isn't that what Brits called television? The *telly?*

Farthing walked dazedly back to his trailer. His mind swarmed. This sudden matter was absolutely intriguing, which livened him up, but on the other hand, it bothered him in a way that could only be called grotesque. Too many coincidences had stacked up too fast. Women selling blood? Old Polaroids of prostitutes? And the old television? At first, he could've sworn that the television had been working last night, showing the most atrocious acts.

But, no. That was impossible. It had been just one nightmare running into the other. The TV could not possibly work.

Infuriated with himself, he shoved the thoughts from his head, mounted the short steps, and entered the trailer. When he pulled the knob to, he winced, for there was still a throbbing ache where he'd cut his finger last night. *What a fuckin' day this crap-sack turned out to be …*

Inside, he detected the stale pipe smell imbued in the walls. But then he noticed another, much more pleasant scent, like soap or shampoo. *Eldred must have one of those plug-in air freshener things, he guessed. He made more contemplations about the mysterious "Piss Car Lady" when he turned down the hallway and made a disconcerting observation. Whereas last night he*'d seen the pale white light flickering in the gap beneath the door to the television room—

What the …

—tonight he noticed the flickering in the gap beneath the *bathroom* door.

I must've left that light on, he surmised but …

Just as he opened the bathroom door, a figure was exiting and bumped right into him. "Who the hell!" he yelled, and at the same time, the figure screamed.

Farthing's no-so-young heart skipped beats; his adrenaline dumped. He knew there was an intruder in his trailer and that meant danger. He stepped back into the hall, was about to flee, but then he took a closer look at the figure.

The figure was a woman, a *nude* woman, and in all, a particularly *attractive nude woman. When she'd bumped into Farthing, she'd been wrapping a towel around her wet hair, having just taken a shower.*

"You scared me sure as fuck gormless!" she yelled in the expected British accent. "Who are you?"

"I might ask you the same question, since you *don't* live here."

Her nudity blared in the harsh fluorescent light, dark cleat-like nipples on small tight breasts looking at him like accusatory eyes. Her still-wet hair betrayed exotic highlights of red, blue, yellow, and green.

"Oh, you must be the American nephew, here for a visit." Her eyes beamed along with a perfect white smile. "It's amazing how much you look like Eldred."

"So I've been told." Farthing tried to recover from his fright and display an appearance of authority and command, but that didn't work so well given the level of distraction her sleek body presented to him. "I, um—well. Who ..." he began, but he was helpless; her raw sexual beauty raved to the extent that he couldn't *not look at her. So—*

Fuckin'-A ...

—so he looked at her.

This vision of her seemed almost electric. Hourglass shape, almost no body fat, toned arms and legs, a flat stomach. South of the belt there was nary a hair. A curious tattoo seemed to arch above her pubis, but the area was too ill-lit to see what it was. Next, his eyes focused on her breasts. Not large but exotically delineated, like firm fruit. They were chiffon-white, with very dark pink-brown nipples pointing straight out. It was utterly arousing: the stark contrast of her nipples against the lambent white of her breasts. And now he noticed this same contrast at her pubis, which was just as white but sided by panty-lines of nut-brown. She must be well acquainted with tanning salons, for these were *preeminent* tan lines.

I give up, he thought. "What was I saying? Oh—who are you? How did you get in here? This is private property, and the door was locked."

Now she was starting to look confused; her calves flexed when she stood on tiptoes as if to look past Farthing over his shoulder. "I guess Eldred didn't mention me. I'm … a friend of Eldred's. Where is he? Just you ask him, and he'll set you to rights."

Farthing had to *force* himself not to imagine sucking those dark, delectable nipples, which looked hard as gumdrops. Finally, his concentration reordered itself. "My Uncle Eldred died recently, I'm sorry to say.

At once, her shoulders dropped, and her vibrant expression collapsed to one of indubitable shock; tears welled instantly in her eyes. "Oh, no—oh my God. It-it can't be," and then she trudged forward, eyes wide in shock, and squeezed past him into the living room.

Whoever she was to Eldred, it must've been significant; this news left her utterly broken up. Farthing followed her erotic soap scents and sat down next to her on the couch. "I'm sorry to offer such bad news, but after all, he'd lived much longer than most; he was close to a hundred, according to his lawyer."

She nodded, sniffling, her face in her hands; as she leaned over, the image of her firm cupcake breasts only distracted Farthing more, which made him feel ashamed. *She's obviously in mourning, and look at me, the scumbag eyeballing her tits …*

"I know, I know," she sobbed. "It's just that …

he had so much vitality. I guess I took it for granted; I guess I thought he'd live forever …"

When Farthing draped a consoling arm about her shoulders, she jerked over closer to him. Farthing didn't know how to put forth the next question without seeming insensitive, but, "But still, miss, I need to know who you are and why you're here. So, my uncle gave you a key to this trailer?"

She nodded again, trying to recompose herself. "I-I'm sure you've put two and two together by now," she began, "but you must understand, Eldred was far more than a client, he was also a very good friend. I adored that man. He helped me out so much when … things went all off track. I could walk in here all down in the dumps, and a minute later, he'd have me happy again and larfin' me arse off."

A … client? Farthing thought, then his stupidity hit him in the head. "Oh, so you're a …"

Finally, she sat back upright and laughed. "I'm a call-girl, a'course. When you walk in your place and find a naked girl standing there, you know I ain't the maid."

Farthing was waylaid. *How do you like that? A whore. And a GREAT LOOKING whore. Even almost a hundred, and Uncle Eldred was still sowing his oats.*

Now, very nonchalantly, she put her arm around him, and her free hand landed on his thigh. In a second, Farthing was erect. He struggled for small-talk. "I see. So-so, how did you first meet Eldred?"

"Oh, he walk into the shop I was workin', 'least ten years ago, and we hit it off right then 'n' there. Guess I was just his type, and that's my good luck, lemme tell ya. After our first session, of course, I let him know that we make house calls to clients we especially like, and that was that. Every two or three months, see, he'd have me come 'ere to stay a week, and we'd have the jolliest time, we would. Any bird in this bizz'll tell ya, most johns are arseholes and bonks, and we gotta pretend that we like 'em. But it weren't nothin' like that with Eldred. He was just fun to be 'round. Hell, I'd probably've come even if he *didn't* have money pourin' out his bum." She relaxed now and put her sleek bare legs up on the coffee table.

Farthing cringed when she leaned over, accentuating the perfect cupcake breasts and exorbitant nipples. His eyes held wide on her curvations until his focus returned.

"I guess you've seen this, right?" she asked with a lascivious grin, and picked up the Polaroid album.

"Um, yes I did ..."

"I'm in it, you know."

Farthing stalled. "I really only flipped through it," he admitted. "Let's see your picture."

She laughed and flipped through some of the higher pages. "Here we are."

Farthing stared. Four different Polaroids were attached to the single page. First was the girl in full-on dominatrix garb, complete with six-inch heels and a black whip, but this was a fetish syndrome Farthing had never found interesting. Two more pics displayed the girl in rather lewd, spread-legged poses. In one, her neck was craned as she sucked her own nipple. In the pic next to it, the girl very dexterously worked a vibrator into her sex, nearly all the way, her entire body glazed in sweat and tensed up, apparently in the throes of climax. The final picture showed only the girl's tight abdomen, glittering with lines of semen that looked like fat slug trails.

Farthing chuckled. "For an old man, Uncle Eldred was certainly virile."

"You ain't kiddin', love, and hung like a horse. That man, I swear, he could go three, four times a day if he'd a mind to it."

The observation only inspired jealousy to Farthing.

However, this photo demonstrated a more

legible view of her rather extensive tattoo, which seemed to be comprised of a long, black spread-winged bat, from hip to hip. "Interesting tattoo," he said, "and a bit sinister."

She laughed. "Yeah, I guess the Goth never wore off of me."

There was also a tiny serpent around her navel. The peek at this invariably dragged his gaze down to the perfectly formed vulva. Farthing could only hope that his erection wasn't obvious. But it wasn't until then that he noticed a scribbled date on the page—nearly a decade ago—and also the cursive word *Mal.*

He hadn't even thought to ask her name. "Is that your name? Mal?"

"That it is …"

"For Mallory?"

"No," she corrected. "Malison. My mother always called me Mal"—another giggle—"said it meant bad in French or Italian or something."

"Well, Mal, I'm pleased to officially meet you. Just called me Farthing." Farthing was trying his best to keep his eyes off her breasts. "And this'll sound odd, but I never even met Eldred and I only spoke to him on the phone a few times when I was just a kid. Nevertheless, he saw fit to make me his sole heir. I couldn't be more grateful for that. My life changed completely."

"Lucky you. Like winning the pools."

"*Pools?*"

"Pools. You know. I guess the lottery's what you Yanks call it …"

Farthing reflected on that. "Yeah, I won the lottery, all right. It's great. But I've only been here two days, and I'm starting to discover … some oddities."

She recrossed her ankles on the coffee table, the movement of which pressed her bare thigh against his own thigh. He had no choice but to gaze down her long legs. It was a *liquid* sight, which his eyes drank in. *Holy shit* … A week ago, the idea that he'd be sitting next to a beautiful nude woman with multi-colored hair was … well. Beyond any mode of conception.

"Tell me about the odd stuff?" she asked.

Where to start? "Well, I heard that Uncle Eldred was in some kind of a club."

"A *club?*" She laughed. "Maybe a *drinking* club."

"Could be, but I think it was more like an alumni club. I heard he went to Cambridge a long time ago. But weirder than that is the people in this club are or were mostly foreigners and they were all very wealthy. Which doesn't make a lot of sense. Why would very rich people hang out with a guy in his nineties who lived in a trailer?"

"You got me, hon. First I've 'eard of it."

"And they all drove very expensive sports cars—I mean, *really expensive*—and the thing is, since I first set foot in this place, I've been seeing a lot of very expensive cars sort of idling around my trailer. I'm talking Rolls Royces, Lamborghinis, like that. Why would people that loaded be looking over an old unit in a *trailer park?*"

"Well, Eldred weren't one to show off, you know? But he was very rich too. I think he just lived here to be inconspicuous."

"But *why?*" Farthing leaned over and emphasized. "Why be inconspicuous? Why be rich but not even own a car or a nice house?"

Mal smiled at him intently. "My, you certainly are curious, ain't ya? But why worry about it? You got it all now. If I was you, I'd be doing bloody handstands in the street."

She's right, he realized. Maybe Farthing was putting too much into the matter because …

Because I got nothing else. Nothing much else in my life … "Okay, I see your point but … But there's another thing. Since I got here, I've gotten several phone calls from people with foreign accents. I thought at first they were telemarketers, but as it turns out, they weren't selling anything. All they did was ask me odd stuff, like, they asked me if I'd been having dreams. One of them told me 'Mind your dreams.' Tell me *that's* not fucked up."

"Sure can't tell ya otherwise, but it's nothin' to go off your rocker about, is it?" She blinked. "It's funny, though, I mean about dreams. Just about any time I'd spend the night here, I'd have me a awful set of nightmares, like, the worst stuff I could imagine. I mean, they was so bad I couldn't even *tell* you."

Farthing contemplated her response in wide-eyed silence. Finally, here was something relative. His own dreams since he'd been here were the worst of his life, the most atrocious things.

She was smiling again, right at him; she squeezed his thigh. "Ya look like you seen a ghost."

When his daze cleared, he found himself looking again—but not on purpose—at her bare pubis. "Not a ghost. Just my own nightmares, now that you mention it. In fact, I even dreamed that that old television in back was on and I was watching it. I mean, it was so realistic that, at first, I thought it was for real, that the TV was *really* turned on, and-and—"

"That old telly, you say? He told me he only had it 'cos it were an antique. It didn't work. But you say it was on?"

"No, I meant I dreamed it was on—I mean, I must have because there's no power cord."

"What was on the screen?" she asked with an increasing interest.

"The worst shit imaginable, like I said. Murder, torture." His belly flip-flopped. "Fuck, it was nauseating. I don't even know how my subconscious mind could come up with stuff like that ... or why ..." But then he remembered the final thing. "Oh, yeah! And I saw this old woman outside tonight, right before I came in. A very *old woman who said her name is Eloise. Do you know anything about her? Did Eldred ever mention her to you?*"

Mal looked right at him, bewildered, and shook her head no.

"She said she's known Eldred for decades, that they were friends, but she also implied that—"

"Let me guess, love. She was a hooker?"

"Well, yes, but like a really long time ago."

Mal nodded, amused. "Hate to spoil your idea of Eldred, but he was a bigtime john, he was. Just about any female friend he ever had was a hooker. He weren't interested in holdin' hands in the park. He'd get right down to the business."

"Yes, yes, I understand that," Farthing hurried on, "but this woman, this Eloise, she said there were occasions when Eldred and his friends would *buy her blood* from her."

Now Mal made a face denoting hilarity. "And she said Eldred slept in a coffin, right?"

"I'm serious! She said these people paid her to take her blood!" Farthing exclaimed.

Now Mal was toying with him. "Did she say *why* these *people bought her blood?*"

"Well—just my luck—no. But she *did* say it was needed by Eldred. She said Eldred had special talents—"

Mal made a high laugh. "Eldred had a special talent, all right. It was in his pants."

Farthing smirked. "According to Eloise, Eldred *showed* all these rich people things."

"He showed the rich people things? What things?"

"I-I don't know. But I think it has something to do with blood. Look, I know it sounds crazy but … Wait! Come here," and then he grabbed her wrist, pulled her up, and led her into the back room.

He flicked on the dim overhead light.

"And there it is," Mal said, still rather mockingly, "the infamous telly that can't be turned on because it ain't got no power cord."

Farthing opened the side drawer. *Let's see what she says about this,* and then he pulled out one of the transfusion bags, some IV lines, and a set of sterile needles. "If you don't believe me, then how do you explain this stuff?"

Suddenly she looked flummoxed, and she walked over. Her nude body was back-lit now, like a cut-out shape, her curves and lines razor sharp. The image was so intensely erotic that Farthing nearly forgot what he was doing …

She took the transfusion bag and stared mystified at it. "Why, of all the jove things, you're right. Bags, needles, the works. All the times I been 'ere, and all the time I spent with Eldred, he never once mentioned anything about health problems or needin' transfusions."

Farthing stepped closer, trying to keep his eyes off her body. Instead, he soaked up the vibrant colors of her still-wet hair and the delicate slope of her throat. "But that's just it. According to his lawyer, he *didn't have health problems, didn't need dialysis or transfusions or anything of the kind. So that just takes us back to what Eloise said: that Eldred needed blood for some reason that* involved all those rich friends of his. She said Eldred had a special *talent* for something."

Mal just looked back at him and shrugged. "Don't know what to tell ya, love. Like we say here in the UK, I think you're floggin' a dead horse. The only one you could ask is dead."

Farthing frustratingly exhaled. Then he turned around to put the transfusion bag, etc., back in the drawer.

Then he stiffened up at a sudden shock.

"Don't worry, I don't bite," Mal said.

She'd stepped right up behind him, grabbed his hips, and roughly pulled him against her. Her hands deftly slid up his front, then slid back down and began smoothing around his crotch.

"Mmm," she whispered. "Feels like something's goin' on down here," and then she gave him a firm, deliberate squeeze.

Shit, he thought in shock. What am I gonna do?

Farthing was long out of practice for this sort of thing. He couldn't have been more uncomfortable, but … some other more primitive instinct seemed to be percolating. His cock was achingly hard, thumping, and drooling in his pants. He could feel her nipples pressed against his back, hard as hot pebbles, and without forethought, he'd already reached one hand behind himself, patted down her delectably warm belly until he found the groove of her sex.

"That's the spirit," she giggled.

What now? She wasn't doing this for her health; she'd expect to be paid. His thoughts scrambled for the right words. "Damn, Mal. You're one of the hottest women I've ever seen—"

"Thank you," she said and kiss his cheek.

"—but I'm an old man out of my league, and I fully get it that you need to be paid for your time, but—"

"Listen to you, dancing around the subject," she laughed. Now one of her hands slid down his pants and was fiddling with his raw cock. "Eldred always paid per quarter, in advance. This is already covered, love."

Oh, fuck. Looks like I'm getting laid …

She unbuckled his pants and had his cock and balls out like magic. She squeezed his shaft, and he felt an abundance of drool pour out. "Yeah, I'm afraid this poor guy needs some attention and fast, eh? Bet you haven't had yourself an oil change in a while," and then she turned him around in place and began to haul him downward.

He nearly thunked to the carpet, his eyes wide in wonder and crude anticipation. When she got him down on the floor, his cock was thumping ludicrously in the air, which seemed to amuse her.

"Just you lay back and let Mal show you how it's done …"

145

The black void seemed to exist in infinite depths, across which drifted skeins of dark-gray smoke; it was a storm of sheer *blackness*, foul odors like burning sulphur, charred woods, and something meaty, like pork.

Next, the vision changed, and he—whoever *he* really was—saw a figure in a cinderblock room lifting other figures—figures tied up in white bundles, mummy-like—and tossing them effortlessly into the open maw of a great roaring furnace. But the parcels—the mummies—were moving, twitching, alive, and through their sackcloth coffins, they screamed in a unison of soul-flaying, ear-rupturing shrieks that seemed to echo without termination. The first figure, the crematorist, at last revealed himself—or *it*self— to be something only vaguely anthropomorphic, more like a vermiculated corpse with a body like a skeleton covered with raw chicken skin, claw-hands with three fingers each, and eyes like sockets filled with pus. Horns sprouted from its anvil-shaped head, and it grinned over rows of teeth like needles of broken glass as it heaved yet another convulsing "mummy" into the furnace.

Other sights blundered into the scope of this cacodemoniacal landscape. Next, a winding country road was seen on a tranquil spring day. In the distance stood a stately fortress, castle-like, but there was an anomaly about the road leading up to the structure. Where most roads in a locale such as this might be lined on either side by well-cut fieldstone fencing, *this* road was lined by rotting corpses stacked five feet high on either side. No army was likely ever to venture up this road, unless they wanted to contribute more building material to the fence.

Next, what dissolved into view was a quiet one-story house in whose backyard stood a six-foot-high dog pen. The pen's interior was empty, though obvious old bloodstains decorated the pen's cement pavement, along with a few bare bones. But handcuffed to the outside of the pen was a hysterical naked woman. She was shapely, attractive, but *worn out.* Bloodshot eyes stared out over the gag in her mouth.

Three men faced her. Two were in dress shoes and slacks, and white dress shirts rolled up at the sleeves; one was short and wiry, another brawny. A third man stood farther back; he had long curly hair, wore jeans and a black t-shirt that read VAN DER GRAFF GENERATOR, and he held a substantial movie camera.

The brawny man finnicked with dials on a high wheeled device from which sprouted two battery cables. One cable had already been clamped to the unfortunate gagged woman's right nipple.

"God*damn*, Knuckles!" complained the shorter man, in a Brooklyn accent. "Can you *believe* Perotti would lie to the boss like that? What is *wrong* with people, huh?"

"Don't know, Roc," replied the brawny man. "Can't figure it. Perotti was set up sweet, but then he pulls a move like *that?*" He looked morosely at the woman hanging on the fence. "Kind of feel sorry for the wife, though, 'cos she's gotta pay the bill."

The shorter man seemed overly agitated. "Aw, *fuck* her, Knucks!," and then—WHAP!—he briskly kicked the woman between the legs. "It's always a woman fuckin' up a guy's life, suckin' his blood dry!" Then—WHAP!—another hard kick. The woman jerked in place, mewling. "Bet she knew *all about* it! Bet she knew Perotti was skimmin' us all along—shit, she was probably *eggin' him* on ta do it just so's she could have herself a new Cadillac!"

The woman's face was beet-red; she was shaking her head *no no no*, but then—WHAP!—another hard kick.

"Damn it, Knuckles! I'm so pissed I'm in a swivet!" The short man then glared at the woman. "Turn that thing on and get with it, will ya? I want this bitch lit up."

"Sure thing, Roc," said the brawny man, then he flicked a toggle on the device, and there was a deep resonant hum.

Meanwhile, the shorter man turned to the guy in the black t-shirt. "Listen, kid. You can probably tell, I ain't in a good mood, so don't fuck this up."

"N-no, sir," said the kid.

"The boss wants close-ups, high-angle shots, and all that good shit, just like fuckin' whatshisname— Hitchcock. Got it?"

"Oh, yes, sir. No problem."

"So get to it. The boss wants good footage, and if it ain't good, we're gonna take your *other* ball." Then he turned back to the nude woman hanging on the fence. "This is gonna hurt a *lot,* sweetie. Then we're gonna show the film to your piece 'a shit hubby, and what we do to him'll be a *hundred times worse,*" and then he turned back to the big man and said, "Let 'er rip!"

When the big man touched the other battery clamp to the woman's left breast, her whole body jerked hard on the fence, and the sound that struggled to issue from behind the gag was like a great muffled *chirp.* Next, the clamp was touched against her bare armpit, and she jerked harder, and now that quick vocal chirp sounded like rocks grinding. As these ministrations ensued, the kid with the camera roved all round the action.

"The pussy now, Knucks," ordered the short man. "Get that clamp right up in there against her pussy—"

"Knucks" wasted no time in executing the command. The edge of that copper clamp was pressed hard up against the woman's tender vulva, and then her body jerked once and then *bowed* against the fence. She just shivered there then, and there was now a sizzling sound, and an aroma drifted about, quite like Spam.

"How do ya like that?" enthused the short man. "Now we know what cookin' pussy smells like."

But then another smell insinuated itself: the remarkable stench of burning hair, because by now, the shivering woman's pubic hair withered and smoked right off her crotch.

The kid with the camera knelt for the close-up.

The short man laughed. "How's that feel, toots? Okay, Knucks. Do the ears now. This is startin' ta get boring."

The woman was still jiggling on the fence with some remnant of life. Knucks put one clamp on her right ear, then—

"That's what I call fuckin' up her day!" celebrated the short guy.

—the other clamp on her left ear, and she flipped and flopped where she hung, and her eyeballs half came out of her head, and she gargled more muffled screams, and then—

POOF!

—all the hair on her head went up in flames, crackling.

"Hot damn!" yelled the short man in glee.

"Yeah, that's really something, Roc." Knucks clicked the machine off and looked upward. The plume of smoke coming off the woman's head looked like something that should come out of a chimney. "Yeah, the boss'll really like this."

The short man clapped. "Okay, kid. Cut."

The kid lowered his camera and smiled. "That's a wrap."

By now, these phantasmal snippets of horror began to assume an identity with regard to their beholder—of course, it was Farthing, and of course, Farthing knew that he must be having more nightmares. But why this plague of atrocious dreams *now* all of a sudden? His soul or the core of his being or whatever the vessel was that provided the abode for his mental self felt buoyant and unfettered, floating in circles in some jet-black abysm that almost reminded him of a turnstile or a revolving door that, every so often, stopped to eject him into a different and previously unseen horror. In other words, Farthing had no arms or legs—he didn't seem to have *any* manner of physical body, but instead, he was propelled along like a balloon in a breeze, and whenever his travels stopped, he found his consciousness sitting in the middle of another visual atrocity.

Sitting *helpless,* that is. Unable to exit. Unable to escape. It was almost like some *other* consciousness were orchestrating this and was *controlling each vision Farthing was forced to watch. One revolting horror after another. The worst things he could ever conceive, or anyone* could ever conceive. In the grips of this … mental abduction, Farthing wanted to scream, but he could not. Instead, he was forced to watch still more …

Now his vision floated about the deck of an old corvette-style ship, not very large and splotched with great patches of rust. Shirtless Black men with rifles milled about the deck, all yakking in whatever language it was they spoke. But then screaming was heard when a large deck-hatch was thrown open, as more armed men dragged up a horde of naked or near-naked Asian people, mostly women and children, all screaming, all crying. Many had been beaten, sporting broken limbs and faces with eyes gouged out. First, a dozen or so were brought up, and one, an elderly man, had his throat cut quickly to the bone, and he was held upside-down over the side so that his blood would spill into the ocean. In less than five minutes, the water surrounding the ship was brimming with sharks.

Screams wheeled up into the cloudless sky as each member of this pitiable naked horde was thrown overboard. With each human parcel dropped into the sea, the shirtless men grinned over the side to watch. Once all the adults had been thrown in, the screaming children went next—

splash! splash! splash!

Most bodies were taken apart piece by piece, as if the sharks were making a sport of this feeding frenzy; some of the smaller children were swallowed whole. Meanwhile, the shirtless spectators all chuckled and grinned in unison

A moment later, the babies were brought up from the hold …

splash! splash! splash!

Farthing thought he could hear his teeth chattering even though he understood that he *had no teeth, no, not in this state of existence. Please, God,* he prayed to the God he'd never believed in, *just let me die right now! I can't hack it! Why are you making me see this shit?*

God, evidently, was not inclined to respond

today.

"Aw, fuck it! Who the fuck cares anyway?" a voice boomed. "The brass doesn't care, so why should we? Fuck it!"

What the hell is THIS now? he wondered, still nauseated from the previous display. The scene had transposed to an expanse of scrubby farmland and some crude fences enclosing pigs and chickens. In the background stood rows of straw-roofed huts, and before the huts stood a wearied congregation of Vietnamese peasants and their ragged families. Each member of the group had eyes glittering with unadulterated hatred. US infantry troops peppered the area surrounding all this, dawdling about with grenade-laden flak vests and black rifles.

One helmeted soldier sat on a tree stump, laughing but with tears in his eyes. "I'm short and we gotta do *this?*" he yelled upward.

Another troop with sergeant stripes looked down. "Come on, L-T. You're platoon leader ... so make the call. The S-3 says the kids are all sappers and the adults are spies for NVA and VC."

Then the man on the stump quickly jumped up, craze-eyed, hysterical. "Yeah, fuck 'em, man! Fuck this shit! This is why they sent me to West Point? Open fire!"

And then machine-guns kicked in, dumping

bullets from all directions into the cluster of civilians, men, women, and children alike. The sound of screams merged with the gunfire to produce a cacophony of madness.

When all the civilians were downed, someone yelled, "Light 'em up!" and a soldier with a flamethrower stepped forward and covered the twitching human pile with roaring fire, then sprayed the huts too. Minutes later, the troops were withdrawing as the entire village released something akin to a black rising mushroom cloud.

"Yeah, fuck it, man!" croaked the lieutenant. "Fuck this shit!"

The last thing Farthing saw were two still-living figures cocooned in flames, trying to stagger away, and that's when Farthing regained consciousness, if it could even be called that, and found himself sprawled out on the carpet of the back room with his shirt pulled open and his pants down, but in spite of this ludicrous position, he felt his heart palpitating, short of breath, and he was vaguely convulsing. There was an awful, rusty taste in his mouth. In fact, he lay there several minutes before he noticed details of his surroundings. One, Mal lay atop him, collapsed as well, her head in his bare lap staring upward and breathing exertedly. Two, the old television was on …

All that the strange circular screen displayed was soundless white static.

What's going on?

He joggled his thighs around in attempts to shake her awake, but she remained there as if paralyzed, face staring upward, eyes open, nipples sticking straight up. "Hey! Mal!" he barked. "Wake up! What's going on?" But it was then that he inadvertently looked to his right and—

His heart nearly stopped.

Standing to the side of him was a young naked girl with long blond pig-tails and small breasts. She stared blankly back at him with bright blue eyes. She couldn't have been more than sixteen years old.

"Who-who are you?" came his very parched question.

The young girl spun around and dashed out of the room.

I must still be dreaming, he thought, and it was a relieving thought, but then Mal was still lying half-across him, naked. "Mal! Damn it! Wake up!"

Finally Mal roused; she sat up, looked around, then looked down at Farthing, her mouth hanging open.

"Mal!" Farthing yelled again. "Why was that girl here?"

"Girl?"

"There was a young blond girl standing here a minute ago, then she ran away. She was *naked*, for shit's sake. Who was she? She looked sixteen years old!

Mal reappropriated some of her sentience, then chuckled. "Her name's Karen. She's one of the group's kids—a little hellion. And I hate to tell you this, but she's *fourteen*."

Farthing bellowed, "What the HELL was she doing here?"

"You probably won't have to worry about it," Mal said, "unless you're a lot dumber than I think. Karen's sort of an insurance policy."

"What the FUCK are you talking about!" Farthing bellowed again. "And, look! The fuckin' TV's on!"

She gazed up at the fizzing screen. Seconds later, it faded off.

Now Farthing was getting the grim idea that this was no dream … "What was on that screen?" he demanded and sat up.

"Oh, it was gorgeous." She seemed like she was in a trance. "You were probably dreaming the same things …"

"What are you talking about?"

"Soldiers," she droned, "shooting civilians.

And-and, Somali pirates, I guess, throwing kids to sharks." She blinked repeatedly. "Some naked woman—getting electrocuted …"

Farthing's head was spinning. "You're right, I *did* dream that, but you saw the same thing on the TV?"

She nodded dopily. "On the telly, yeah." And then she rubbed her face in her hands. "That's how it works. It's been so long since I've gotten to see it …"

"See *what?*" he snapped.

She kind of sidled over then, grinning inanely. "If I told you, you wouldn't believe it."

Farthing pulled his pants back up, rebuttoned his shirt. The inside of his mouth tasted so rank, he actually expectorated against the wall. *Fuck it!* Then he looked down at Mal again and noticed a scabbed cut on her arm with some dried blood showing. "What did you do? You cut yourself?"

Mal giggled lazily. "Trust me. You wouldn't believe any of it if I told you … It's the kind of thing where … you can't be *told*. You have to be *shown* …"

This was infuriating; he hated feeling out of control. Something was way, way wrong here, and he knew that she was stringing him along. "Who are you really? My uncle's call-girl? Bullshit!"

"Well, you might say I'm all that and more. Oh, and you and I? We fucked twice, by the way. You did pretty good for an old man—you came like a champ!"

Farthing wanted to grab her by the throat and shake her, *make* her tell him the truth. But when he reached out to do just that—

"Oww!"

Somebody behind him grabbed him by his hair and twisted.

Who the fuck!

Farthing was raised to his feet by his hair. When he was able to collect his faculties, he saw that two men had entered the room, two men in suits, and that's when Farthing's heart began to trip. *It's some kind of a shake-down,* he guessed. *The bitch set me up for a robbery!* But then …

The two intruders didn't look like robbers. One was short, sixtyish, with short gray kinky hair; he looked Middle-Eastern. A genuine Rolex adorned his left wrist. The other man, the one who'd lifted Farthing by his hair, was considerably larger—six-five at least, longish black hair, a great wedge for a face, and a football-player's physique. He released Farthing and stared blankly at him with one eye; the other eye was covered by an eyepatch.

"Pardon our unexpected intrusion, Mr.

Farthing," said the man with the Rolex in a clipped Arabic accent. "My name is Saed, and the refrigerator-sized gentlemen to your right is Walter. You've already made acquaintance with our—shall we say—our operative, Mal, and you've already sampled firsthand the only thing she's good for."

"Thanks a lot," Mal replied, smirking up.

"You see, Mr. Farthing," this Saed continued, "we use Mal as a gatherer of intelligence, you could say. Before we could proceed—since your good uncle is regrettably no longer among the living—we needed to ascertain just how much you know. What I mean is, how much of the process your uncle divulged to you. But according to our slatternly friend Mal, the answer to that question is exactly nothing. Is that correct?"

"He don't know shit," Mal said, finally getting up off the floor. Her skin looked yellowy in the dim light. "And can ya believe it? He never even *met* Eldred. How fucked up is that?"

Saed grinned modestly at her. "Not nearly as fucked up as *you're* going to be if you don't manage to get yourself pregnant and keep it this time."

Mal's expression darkened. "I got two nuts out of him; that's a good start, ain't it?"

Farthing bellowed, "What the fuck are you

talking about? How much of the process my uncle divulged to me? How much of *what process? And you want Mal pregnant?* With *my kid? What the fuck for?"*

Saed turned toward Mal. "I'll need a word or two in *private* with Mr. Farthing, if you please. Run along now and join Asenieth and Kirill in the living room." He smiled thinly. "I'm sure they'll find something productive for you to do. And go with her, Walter."

The big man with the eyepatch nodded, then nudged Mal out of the room.

"You're the people who've been calling me," Farthing snapped, "and driving around here in expensive cars."

"Oh, but of course, but there are many more of us than you've seen. We're testing the waters; like I said, we needed to know what Eldred may have told you, if anything."

Farthing was steaming. "And what the hell was that naked girl doing in here?"

"Merely an inducement, Mr. Farthing. Our dear little Karen will serve well should you choose not to cooperate." Saed took out his cellphone and showed Farthing some pictures on it.

And here was Farthing, lying on the floor with his pants down as the naked blond girl lay next to him. Next, Farthing's hand on her bare breast. Next, his hand between her legs.

"That's bullshit!" Farthing yelled. "I never touched her! I was asleep since the minute I came back here with Mal!"

Saed's brow popped up. "I'm afraid these snapshots beg to differ. It would be bad news for you, Mr. Farthing, if these pictures ever found their way into the hands of law enforcement, don't you think?"

"You motherfuckers are setting me up!" Farthing knew now. "Why? For my uncle's money?"

At this suggestion, Saed laughed. "That's hardly likely, since your uncle's fortune actually came from our little group. What you're failing to understand is that we *need* you, Mr. Farthing. It works out better for everyone if you play along, and when you realize the extent of the situation here, you'll *want to go along.*"

Farthing's confusion left him to stand in silence as Saed turned his back and bent to visually peruse the old television. He placed his hand on top of it. "Hmm, still warm."

"And what the FUCK is with that television? It was on a few minutes ago, Mal was watching it—"

"But you were asleep, yes? Were you dreaming the same things that Mal saw on the screen?"

"Yes! And that's crazy!"

Saed turned back to look at Farthing. "Oh, it's more than crazy, Mr. Farthing, and it's also proof of the purity of your line."

Farthing's entire face creased. "My *line?*"

"Your *bloodline,* which is clearly the same as Eldred's. It's *complicated,* Mr. Farthing, and you'll need some time to acclimate to the truth of things. Now, you think this old television along with the things you've witnessed are *crazy?* Well, how's *this* for crazy? Your Uncle Eldred comes from a long hereditary line of warlocks—"

"Give me a break, you fuckin' *crackpot!*" Farthing yelled back. "You're full of shit!" He paused, squinted, then began laughing out loud. "My uncle was a warlock, huh?"

"Yes," Saed informed him, "and so are you."

Farthing could feel his face turning red.

"You're the same stock, Mr. Farthing. We know that because you've been having the dreams— dreams that your own subconscious couldn't possibly concoct on its own. You would never believe it if I told you, so let's not waste time. I'll *show* you." Then he walked to the doorway. "Mal? Walter? If you will?"

Mal remained unabashedly naked; she was holding, of all things, a plastic cup. Meanwhile,

Walter took the chair that was leaning against the back wall, unfolded it, and set it in front of the television.

"Have a seat, Mr. Farthing," Saed said.

Farthing smirked at all of them. "No."

Saed's eyes widened. Mal sighed. And Walter produced a sizable knife.

"What?" Farthing laughed. "You're gonna *kill me* if I don't sit in the chair?"

Saed stared at him. "No, but depending on the extent of your disobedience, you'll likely *wish* you were dead. This means a great deal to us, so, please, Mr. Farthing. Make no difficulties. It will only force us to resort to unpleasant measures."

Mal touched his shoulder. "Do as he says, love. You don't wanna fuck with these people—they're sick in the head. They'll *fuck you up* in ways you can't imagine, but they won't let you die. Take my word for it. You stay on their good side and do what they tell you, and you'll have a very nice life."

Farthing glared at her, at her jutting, tan-lined breasts, then he glared at Saed.

Then he looked at Walter's very sharp knife. Walter seemed to look back more with his eyepatch than with his actual eye.

"The easy way, or the hard way? Why not put your belligerence aside for a few moments and see

164

what we have to offer?"

Farthing sat down in the chair.

"Good! Good!"

But now Farthing was staring in shock at Mal and Walter. Mal had her arm out while Walter, with his knife, made a tiny puncture wound directly under the scab that had already dried.

The obvious pain made her clamp her teeth together. With her other hand, she held the cup and let the blood drip into it. When Walter squeezed her arm, the blood dribbled out faster.

Farthing recalled cutting his finger on something, then sucking the blood off it—immediately before he thought he'd seen the television on. And earlier today, when he'd been dreaming those atrocities, he detected a rank, metallic taste in his mouth, then noticed that Mal had somehow cut herself. It was a very grim *two and two* that he put together …

"Don't think for a minute that I'm gonna drink blood," Farthing said. "*That's* what this is all about? The empty blood-collection bags in the TV stand? And the old woman, Eloise, said Eldred and his 'friends' would pay her for her blood …"

"Eloise?" Saed intoned in surprise. "She's still alive?"

"Been in the booby hatch," Mal said, "but I guess they let the old munter out, and then she got to runnin' her mouth to Farthing here."

Saed smiled at Farthing. "At any rate, Mr. Farthing, you're right, in a sense. It is all about blood, and it always has been, for time immemorial. Or I should say, *sullied* blood, from an unsanctified person—such as Mal, for instance, or Eloise. There's no shortage of such persons: willing to sell their God-given lifeblood for a song."

"The other day I cut my finger and then I licked it," Farthing began. "Then the television came on. So my blood is *sullied too?*"

"Well of course! And just as your uncle before you," Saed said. "The most sullied blood of all. Do you know who Simon Magus was?"

"Fuck no!"

"A sorcerer of nefarious import, I'm afraid. He was known in the first century as the *Bad* Samaritan and the First Heretic. He tried to *buy* his way into Jesus's entourage of Apostles. He could fly in the air, he could levitate his enemies, he could raise the dead and convert base metals into gold, Mr. Farthing, and that's no fairy tale. I'll add that Simon Magus is your and your uncle's lineal forebear."

Farthing was trying to see whatever logic it was that these insane people believed. "And—let me guess—that means that *I* have his powers now. Well, hate to tell you this, but I'm not flying and you sure as shit aren't levitating."

"Not so much his powers, Mr. Farthing, but his potential to solicit *favor*."

Farthing's smirk was starting to feel permanently pressed into his face. "I got no idea what you're blabbering about! You're all nuts!"

Saed smiled. "That's an expected reaction; after all, you're only human. Let's see how you feel once we've concluded out little demonstration." He looked to Walter. "Bring in the others, Walter."

"The girl too?"

"Of course! Karen is as much a part of our fellowship as any of us …"

"That's what you call this?" Farthing complained. "A fellowship? I call it a whackjob cult. Devil worshipers? Really? Warlocks?"

"I'd mind my tongue, Mr. Farthing, until you've seen what we have to show you. I'm in a particularly good mood today. You don't want to see me in a bad one," and then he turned as Walter re-entered the room, followed by the young girl, Karen (who was now dressed), and two more adults.

A very fat man in sports jacket and slacks, with salt-and-pepper hair was introduced as "Kirill, one of the famed Russian oligarchs." He nodded curtly to Farthing. "I'm honored," he addressed Farthing in the Russian accent.

A shapely, sharp-looking woman in her forties or fifties was "Asenieth, quite a powerful woman in the Turkish defense ministry." The woman offered Farthing a licentious smile that sent a chill up his spine. "Meeting you, sir, is such a prestigious event. I only regret that I am too old to bear your children."

Well that's a fine how-do-you-do, Farthing thought. There was something densely alluring about the woman. But a more potent chill went up his spine when he noticed that Karen, the fourteen-year-old, was grinning at him as well, and just once very quickly brushed her hand up between her legs. Farthing felt like he had snakes suddenly churning in his belly.

Saed was grinning. "Mr. Farthing does not believe in the validity of our coterie, nor in the power of his and his uncle's bloodline."

"Then I suggest we remedy that posthaste," said Kirill, and then, from his jacket, he removed a small cocktail fork.

"Fucker!" Farthing yelled; from behind, Walter had instantly put him in a full nelson, and suddenly Farthing was squirming helpless in the chair.

Saed went on, "If you refuse to drink this cup of blood, Kirill will pull your eyeball out of your head with his fork, and if you don't believe he's capable of doing such a thing …"

Again, Saed brought out his cellphone and accessed the video gallery, then held its screen before Farthing's eyes.

Farthing nearly threw up. "You fuckin' psycho pieces of shit!"

The video depicted Kirill slowly digging the eyeball out of a person's skull. The worst part was that the victim was a little girl, even younger than Karen. A shriek like a teapot shot from the phone; Farthing suspected that the sound would haunt him for the rest of his life.

"You sick fucks …" Farthing couldn't even yell anymore.

"So, Mr. Farthing," Saed continued. "What's it going to be?"

The cocktail fork hovered.

"Just do it, Farthing," Mal implored. "These people ain't foolin' around. Don't fuck everything up for yourself. Just … drink it," and then she moved the plastic cup to Farthing's lips.

All forethought seemed to sever in Farthing's head. He was unable to consider what he was about to do.

He just did it.

Mal tipped the cup, filled Farthing's mouth with the blood. He sensed the salty iron burst of unwholesome flavor. Then he grimaced and swallowed.

It was common in the court of Genghis Khan that detractors, captured foreign generals, and enemies of the state be tortured while on display for all the court to see. A beaten, bearded, flea-bitten man was tied up like a long package and lain on his side on a wooden table. A number of Khan's soldiers held the prisoner down tight as a smoking crucible was tipped and then molten lead was poured into the prisoner's ear. The prisoner put up quite a fight, but it didn't take him long to settle down, shivering, as the molten metal poached his brain from the inside out.

Mounted next to him, however, were two wooden posts about four feet apart and six high. Forming a human web, so to speak, between the posts was a naked woman, hung upside-down, her ankles and wrists tied to the posts such that her body formed an X-shape. Her physique tensed and flexed as she bellowed, but alas, the sound of her screams could not be heard. There was only a death-like silence. Two soldiers approached, each holding an L-shaped spoon-like instrument, both of which were inserted into the woman's vagina;

then each man pulled his tool, and this sufficed to open the woman's vagina as far as it could go. Next, another crucible was brought forward by a grim-faced Mongolian metallurgist, only this one was filled with molten *silver,* which had a much higher melting point, and with a consummate skill, he slowly emptied the crucible's contents into the woman's opened sex organ. The look on her face and the tremors of her body defied description, and all the onlookers—including the jewel- and leather-clad man who was Khan himself—watched with smiling satisfaction.

The Comanche Indians were equestrian nomads who believed that the only way to properly defend themselves was to kill all human beings who *weren't* Comanches, not just the English settlers and the Spanish and the French but even other Native American tribes who got anywhere near them, and their expertise at torture was well-honed on white men and Native Americans alike. Would-be settlers would travel across the southern plains only to be greeted by tracts of land upon which men had been stripped and staked to the ground. Their lips, ears, noses, and eyelids were cut off, along with their genitals, those wounds immediately cauterized by torches so the prisoner wouldn't bleed to death, and if that weren't bad enough, the victim was then forced to eat his own raw testicles. This, in other words, was the Comanche calling card: *Come onto our land and this will happen to you.*

Children and women of other tribes were taken as slaves to be worked to death. But children of the white men, and even babies, were fastidiously scalped, for the younger the scalp, the more potent the magic. Infant penises, too, were taken, and added to necklaces for good luck. One Comanche elder, captured by US troops in 1875, possessed a necklace with over one hundred baby penises threaded to it. The most attractive of Caucasian women were raped *en masse* by the tribe's braves but then suffered a fate worse than death when they were thrown to the Comanche *women,* where they'd be slowly tortured for days with bone needles, hot coals, and thorn branches. See, the Comanche women didn't like the idea of these white bitches receiving the seed of their husbands. Less attractive white women had their hands and the soles of their feet burned to the bone, and then they were left alive in the great outdoors, eventually to be eaten by buzzards, coyotes, and mountain cats.

Though the number is likely exaggerated, it's said that King Henry VIII had over 70,000 people executed, and most of these executions were by means of beheading. Through Royal Acts of Attainder, Henry would condemn anyone who so much as whispered words of opposition; some even former best friends, not to mention two of his wives. If Henry didn't like a person's face, then that person was beheaded.

But the famous Tudor king didn't send *all* of his enemies to the headsman; he had a penchant for torture. Henry enjoyed watching prisoners being "pressed" to death, a slow process in which the victim is placed under a wooden board, and upon the board, one at a time, heavy weights were placed. Over time, of course, the bones would snap and internal organs would be squeezed out of orifices.

Henry was also captivated with *boiling* certain offenders alive. The victim—nude, of course—would be hung upside down over a boiling cauldron of water, then lowered, often slowly, until the head was completely submerged. But after a moment, he would be raised back up out of the water. Then, off again, on again, he'd be repeatedly dunked, the body lowered a little more each time. The process would be protracted for as long as the victim was able to retain even the tiniest bit of life. Before the entire body blistered, the skin would take on the hue of raw beef. Or sometimes, when a more expeditious end was ordered by the king, the victim would be fully lowered and held there, flipping and flopping at the end of the rope and screaming under the scalding water until he involuntarily inhaled. Sometimes, Henry's noblemen friends would complain of wives or mistresses who committed infidelities, so Henry would grant these men their vengeance, condemn said wives and mistresses without the benefit of a trial, then have them stripped naked, tied up, and heaved into the cauldron for the husbands to witness along with the king.

The mystical entity known as the "Mob" has demonstrated a formidable diversity when it comes to the disposal of human bodies. New Orleans kingpin Carlos Marcello (who is said to have actually hired the assassins of John F. Kennedy) took great pleasure in welding his enemies into steel drums and leaving the drums to float in the immense swamplands in high summer, where the occupant would essentially be roasted to death, after which the barrel would be sunk by rifle shots. Sometimes, other Mob bosses and "capos" would bring "rats," "snitches," and "stoolies" to Mr. Marcello's estate; their legs would be broken, then they'd be boated out to the swamps and flopped overboard, such that they'd foundered, screaming, in the water. Mr. Marcello and his associates would often smoke cigars, drink, and watch from the boat as the stoolies were chopped up into chunks and swallowed by an eager population of alligators.

Car compactors were another convenient way in which such criminal elements would make bodies disappear, all the more practical since the Mob owned so many junkyards. A stolen car would be filled with dead bodies and then "cubed" in the compactor. And it was not uncommon for this procedure to be implemented when still-*living* bodies were stuffed into the cars.

Also, there are these fascinating industrial machines known variously as "car shredders," "metal shredders," and "cement shredders," and they are absolutely intriguing to watch. The machines can be thought of as giant gear-boxes, whose sprocketed gears are made of super-hard steel alloys. An entire car can be dropped in such a machine, and those intersecting gears will slowly and completely tear it apart, engine block and all. Porcelain toilets and chunks of cinderblock walls can be dropped into the machine and be completely pulverized. Even inch-thick steel plates are fed into the machine and ripped apart an inch at a time, without putting the least bit of stress on the powerplant.

A US construction company left several such shredding machines in Afghanistan when the US military withdrew from that esteemed country; hence, they are now the prized property of the Taliban, who don't use them for shredding steel plates and cars. They use them to shred living human beings.

It was all these things and more that were displayed in living color on the old round-screened television set in the back room.

And Farthing, with his belly full of whore's blood, could only sit there watch while his guests stood behind him and watched as well. They all watched for hours and hours.

Farthing awoke in a tumult of jostling, frenetic movement. He felt a hand at his throat, squeezing, such that he could barely breathe. He felt hot sweat dripping on him and heard someone either moaning in pleasure or gasping in anguish. When he opened his eyes amid the terror, he saw slices and blurs of Mal, tensed and naked, straddling him on his bed. A croaking sound leaked out of his throat, then the hand came off and he could breathe again; at the same time, he felt a dislocated but intoxicating orgasm pulse out of him.

It took him a minute or two to regain his breath and senses. Once again, he found himself in his uncle's big bed with no recollection of getting there. The last thing he remembered was sitting in the back room after having been forced to drink the cup of Mal's warm, coppery blood and then watching that infernal television. And everything he'd seen on the screen he remembered all too well.

He was naked now and sprawled out on the bed like a dropped dummy, and it was Mal, of course, who was straddling him. The slick interior of her vagina seemed to gulp Farthing's limpening cock, coaxing out some last, post-ejaculatory sensations. When he groggily looked up at her, she shined completely, as if she'd been doused in baby oil.

She grinned down. "God*damn*, love. You put most men your age to shame."

"What the fuck have you been doing?" he yelled. "Having sex with me against my will?"

She laughed outright. "First time I've heard a man complain about *that.*"

"And after all that awful shit I saw on the TV, I don't know how I could possibly even get it up ..."

She pointed to the nightstand. There was a little label-less bottle and eyedropper there. "Just a bit of tincture's all that's needed—"

"*Tincture?*"

"Red ginseng oil and goat weed," she said. "It's ancient and it works. It'll put a boner on a dead man. And you got me off twice. Not a lot of men can do that. It was lovely …"

She drugged me and fucked me, came the bald realization. Then he thought, *The television, those people …*

"Must be the situation," she went on, moving some mysterious inner vaginal muscles around his now-deflated cock. "There's just something about *evil* that's very arousing—"

He tried to sit up but wasn't quite able. "*Evil?* Are you shitting me? That's what you think this is? Uncle Eldred was a fuckin' *warlock? So that must make you*—what?—a witch, you and that Turkish nut-job out there? You idiots all think you're worshiping the devil?" He tried to get up again, but her thighs clamped him down. "I guess some people can get so *rich that there's nothing left for them. You can only buy so many* Maseratis before it gets dull. So you convince yourselves that you're servants of Satan, for shit's sake. The new thing to do. Well, let me tell you something—"

She kept grinning down; she tweaked his nipples. "You do that, sweetie. Tell me."

"—there's no such thing as evil. It's just mental illness. It's just people going pure-ass crazy!"

Mal's laughter fluttered upward. "Oh man, you really got a ways to go, ain't ya? I don't know how you can *not* believe now, not after what you saw on the telly."

Farthing grimaced. *The fuckin' TELLY.* "The devil's television set? Is that what you're telling me? What a crock of shit!"

"How *can* it be? We all saw it too—it was glorious. Henry VIII boiling naked chicks alive? Those people in the swamp getting eaten by crocodiles—er, no, alligators, right? The Taliban dropping women and children alive into those crusher machines? How sweet was that? Makes my pussy soak, seeing that. And you get the show every night, with or without the telly. Lucky you. Same bloodline as your uncle. Everything you dream is all from the same source as what you saw on the television."

Farthing just stupidly lay there, locked under her thighs. But what was she saying? What did she mean? She'd seen the same thing he saw on the television, and last night, when they'd fallen asleep on the floor, she'd described the *exact same nightmares* that he'd had.

How could this be possible?

His head was spinning too much to contemplate further.

She jiggled her hips a little. "Feels like your jism's starting to leak out," and then she quickly climbed off and was standing oddly spread legged by the nightstand. He could see a line of his own sperm slowly oozing down the inside of a thigh, then—

"What the *fuck are you doing?*"

—she held a little plastic cup there and let the semen run into it.

"Two birds with one stone, eh?" she said. Now the little cup was half-full of Farthing's sperm. "Can't take any chances this time. Between me and Karen? One of us has *got* to get pregnant by you."

"You're gonna—" His eyes bugged. "She fuckin' *fourteen!*"

"Sure. Had her first period a few years ago, so she's plenty fertile. One of us is bound to get pregnant." She held the little cup up and winked. "I'm gonna go pour this in her pussy, and this is how it'll be till both us are knocked up. Eldred knocked *me* up a few years back, and it looked like everything would be fine, but then ..." She paused a moment and went blank-faced. "I lost it. They were so pissed, I thought sure they'd kill me— thought they were gonna do a skin-job on me. They do that, you know, when people aren't any use to them anymore. It's like I told ya earlier, love.

180

These people aren't foolin' around. Now, take a shower and get dressed. We'll be waiting for you in the living room."

Farthing was too mortified to cogitate all of this at once. When she began to trounce off to the bedroom door, he glanced at the double doors leading out to the short balcony.

Mal didn't have to turn when she said, "And don't even *think* about trying to leave. All they'll have to do is call the police and show 'em those pix of you molesting little Karen and you'll be in the clink in double-quick time. The peddies in there will *love* you."

"I didn't molest anyone!" Farthing yelled. "That was a set up!"

"Right. Take a shower and get dressed," and then she walked out of the room with the little cup of semen.

Farthing's mortification showed no signs of abating as he showered, dressed, and pondered. The fleeting fantasy that he would suddenly awaken from a ghastly dream kept titillating a segment of his consciousness, and the more time that ticked by, the grimmer he felt and the more manifest it became that this was very real and he was in a very deep bind.

He wandered out to the living room. The

television was on—not the one in the back room but a regular big flat-screen television. A local newscaster was prattling away in her expected British accent. Farthing stared at what awaited him.

Walter leaned against the kitchen counter, smoking a cigarette. There was no sign of the little girl, Karen. Saed and Kirill were calmly engrossed in a card game at the coffee table. But right on the floor lay Mal, still naked, squirming in obvious turmoil while Asenieth, with her skirt hiked up, was squatting crudely over her head, sitting on her face.

"Lick up, you dirty cunt," she ordered in a hot whisper. "Do it right!" And at the same time, she very daintily dragged the point of an icepick along the side of Mal's neck. "Do it better, bitch, like last time, or else I'll stick this in your neck and fuck this carpet all up with your whore blood ..."

Just more madness, Farthing thought.

"Ah, Mr. Farthing," said Saed, looking up from his cards with a smile. "I'm glad you decided to join us."

Farthing looked at Walter, grimaced, then asked, "Where's the little girl?"

"She's departed for the night. Her parents just picked her up. But she'll be back tomorrow for another … insemination, if you will."

"Of course, you're welcome to fuck her direct," Kirill said above his huge stomach, "if that's your preference. Believe me, in spite of her age, she's no stranger to a man's love."

Farthing's stomach instantly shimmied. "This is just sheer insanity. What do you hope to gain by this … what is it? A satanic club? You're all play-actors, worshiping the Prince of Fuckin' Darkness?"

Asenieth was squealing now, still sitting on Mal's face with Mal's tongue foraging in her superior's vagina. "Good, good, you little cunt. You're finally getting it right." Then Asenieth waved the icepick. "I should stick this in your nose and smack it back all the way to your brain, bitch. Jiggle it around, just for fun …"

"Please don't do that, dear Asenieth," Saed said with a smile. "We need our good servant Mal, for many things." Then his eyes addressed Farthing. "You see, it's all about producing an heir who will continue to bring forth the dark wonders for all of us to see."

Farthing smirked. "Whatever it is you nut-jobs believe—it's asinine. And you think—what?—using my sperm to knock her or that little girl up will—"

"It will secure the permanence of your

precious bloodline," Kirill said, "that is, your *uncle's bloodline.*"

Saed grinned. "Pardon the pun, but we've had a *devil* of a time getting Eldred to sire a child. Mal lost one, and so did several other women in the past. Perhaps our prayers weren't fervent enough, nor our sacrifices. But they will be this time."

"Wait, look!" Aseneith said excitedly. She pointed to the flat-screen, on which the newscaster rambled on: "… and in news from the coast, an eighty-nine-year-old local woman, Eloise Anstruther, was found dead in her car this morning near Burnstow. Ms. Anstruther was a former mental patient and apparently homeless at the time of her death. The police are classifying her death as a homicide, as her throat had been cut …"

"Are you shitting me?" Farthing complained to his guests. "You murdered that harmless old woman?"

"I wouldn't say harmless as much as *use*less," Saed elaborated. "Walter did the work for us earlier after you had passed out …"

Walter glanced at Farthing, then briefly opened and closed his suit jacket, momentarily showing a very large knife in a scabbard.

"But you can thank yourself in general, Mr. Farthing. When you revealed last night to Mal that

Eloise had been talking to you, well, we couldn't have that. But Eloise was a loyal subject some time ago, I'll give her that."

Jesus, Farthing thought. *If I hadn't brought it up to Mal, the old lady would still be alive.* "So, tell me. She was part of this cult of yours? She was giving you *blood?*"

"Sullied blood, yes, Mr. Farthing. She was once a trusted attendant, and many decades ago, she even became pregnant by Eldred. Like Mal, however, Eloise lost the child early on. We're hoping that *you* will break the previous string of bad luck."

Farthing ground his teeth and rubbed his eyes in frustration. "So … you're telling me that you want *me* to impregnate someone so that the Farthing bloodline can continue?"

"Yes!"

"Why?"

The room fell silent, and the interlopers all looked at each other, smiling. "Because," Saed continued, "you're the only one left alive who can … turn on the television, so to speak," and then he winked.

Farthing stared, his mouth hanging wide. "What exactly *is* that old TV in the backroom?"

"You could call it a mirror, a crystal ball in reverse, you could call it many things. And to those who live to serve our benefactor, you can call it a blessing. What makes the world go round, Mr. Farthing? I'll tell you: money. There are many of us, and we're among the wealthiest people on Earth. How did we get this way?" Saed locked eyes with Farthing. "By faith."

"Faith in the fuckin' *devil?* Are you shitting me? This is a joke, right?"

"Address him by any name you choose," Kirill cut in. "Shaitan, Iblis, Belial, Lord of the Air. The more names, the better. The more titles by which he can be praised. The Morning Star, Apollyon. The Father of the Earth ..."

Saed put down his hand of cards. "I can only imagine your dubiety, Mr. Farthing. You, an empiricist, an atheist. A believer in nothing."

This was, for the most part, true, but Farthing still took offense. "Fuck you. You don't know anything about me or what I believe in."

"You believe in nothing—your *blood* says so. But this time tomorrow, you'll have no choice but to believe." Saed sat back in the plush couch, relaxing. "Let's just pretend for a moment that you were a devout Christian, that you'd fully and honestly opened your heart to Jesus. Wouldn't it be absolutely ecstatic, absolutely enthralling, to be allowed on certain occasions to see what He has seen, with His very eyes? His miracles, His sermons, His turning water to wine? When Jesus told Lazarus to come out of the tomb, Lazarus arose from the dead and came out." Saed's eyes glittered. "Wouldn't a Christian give *anything* to see that? To see what Jesus saw?"

Farthing could fathom no response, except, "The things I saw on that fuckin' television definitely *weren't* the visions of Jesus."

"No, they weren't. They were the visions of someone else. Hence, our coterie, our little group here, formerly empowered by your uncle. Now, we are empowered by you."

"Because one of my ancestors was a *warlock?*" Farthing blurted. "You think I *believe* that? You think I *believe* that that piece of shit television in the back room will only turn on when I drink blood—"

"*Sullied* blood, Mr. Farthing, the blood of those who willingly reject the salvation that Christ's sacrifice offers."

Spittle flew from Farthing's lips. "Bullshit! You expect me to believe that a fuckin' television shows the visions of the *devil?* Bullshit!"

"It's all about faith, Mr. Farthing," Kirill cut in. "Our benefactor rewards the faithful, just as God does. What we all saw previously on the television are visions that no living human beings have *ever* seen. What a privilege that is, no? Isn't it a supreme privilege to be able to see what angels can see?"

"Angels?" Farthing spat. "Don't make me laugh. Torture, brutality, murder? Those are the visions of *angels?*"

"I'm sorry," Kirill corrected. "I meant one angel in particular. Through the mystic wonders of your uncle, we've been blessed, and we will continue to be blessed through you."

"Enough for tonight," Saed said. He stood up, seeming amused. "We'll leave you now, Mr. Farthing, to reckon your future with us and your importance in the midst of this wonder. But we'll be back tomorrow to chat more."

"No hurry. Don't knock yourself out," Farthing said, frowning.

"And just to keep you company, of course, we'll leave Mal and Walter with you."

"Thanks. Thanks a fuck of a lot."

Saed, Kirill, and Asenieth all smiled at Farthing, then filed out of the trailer.

"Fuck," Farthing mumbled. "What a fucked up day."

"It won't take long before you feel differently," Mal offered. "You really are part of something very important."

Farthing grimaced. Meanwhile, Walter opened

the fridge and pulled out a bottle of beer.

"Oh, help yourself to my beer, why don't you?" Farthing sniped.

"It's your uncle's beer," Walter said, "and don't piss me off, mate. I ain't in the mood." Then he scratched his eyepatch, sat down on the couch, lit a cigarette.

"So, what?" Farthing ventured. "You're keeping me prisoner here?"

"I wouldn't quite say that." Walter spewed smoke up toward the ceiling. "You can do what you want, go where you want, but … you know what happens if ya try to give us the slip."

Farthing knew.

He couldn't resist. "Lemme ask you something. Are glasses half price for you—I mean, because you've only got one eye?"

That single eye looked right back at Farthing, and Walter smiled. "You'll get yours, mate. Just you wait."

"Let's go in the bedroom," Farthing said to Mal. "This guy's not exactly the life of the party."

Walter smiled and showed his middle finger. Farthing led Mal to the master bedroom.

"You know, you can put some clothes on if you want," he told her.

Mal shrugged. "They want me to keep you …

interested."

"Ah, yes. So you'll get pregnant and extend the Farthing bloodline …"

"Yeah," she said. "Blokes are all alike. Show 'em a naked bird, and that's all they care about. They let their tallywackers do their thinkin' for 'em."

Farthing opened a window; the day's heat had subsided, and now the nighttime exuded cool air and a distant sound of crickets. For some reason, the crickets sounded different in England. "That may be true, but this is one *bloke* who's had enough sex for the time being. But I'm really curious now. How do you fit into all of this?"

Mal put her bra and panties on, and that was all. She lay down on the bed. "I told ya. Through Eldred. He come into my shop one day, I hauled his ashes a few times, then I started doin' house calls. What can I say? The old bugger liked me, and he was rich. He was a very nice guy, to be honest. One of the few johns I liked bein' around."

"No, I mean—" His hand gestured the direction of the living room. "All *that* business, with *those* people?"

"The group, you mean."

"Yeah, the group."

"They was already up with Eldred, had been for a long time. They knew all about him."

"He was already *up* with a bunch of satanists, you mean?"

"It's not as trivial as you think. These people are for real." She crossed her ankles on the bed, stretched; she seemed very lackadaisical. "The occult, witchcraft, satanists—it all has this hokeyness attached to it. Punk kids from bad families, listening to all that shitty black metal and sacrificing cats and havin' orgies 'n' whatnot. That ain't *these* people, believe me."

"Yeah," Farthing went on. "Those assholes are all nuts; they believe their own delusions. They believe that Satan gave them riches in return for their faith. A bunch of idiots. But you're not like that, right? Sure, you play along when they're around because they pay you. But you seem like the only one of the bunch who's sane."

Mal giggled. "Oh, I'm sane, all right. Sane enough to know what's real when I got my face pushed in it."

What did that mean? "Come on. You don't *really* believe in the devil, do you?"

She looked at him deadpan, her arms folded under her tight bosom.

Farthing frowned. "So you're telling me you truly believe that that old TV in there can show people the visions of the devil ..."

"Not just *any* people," she said, looking off. "Only the select few, and only when triggered by someone from the right lineage. Like you."

Fuck, he realized. *She's insane too.* "Sorry, but I can't buy it. I don't know how they rigged it … The TV must run on batteries, and I guess people that rich could have movies made that looked that authentic."

Mal laughed and shook her head.

"Okay. I'll pretend. Let's say I believe it all. What's the explanation for the TV?"

"The telly?"

"Yeah, the *telly.* Where did it come from? How does it work?"

"No one knows, and Eldred wasn't very talkative about it. He'd only give us little bits and pieces of an explanation. We think he built it himself—"

"That's preposterous," Farthing blurted. "He built a fucking *television* that shows—"

"The most evil events in history, all witnessed through the eyes of Satan himself. Think outside the box, Farthing. You're thinking it's scientifically impossible to build something like that—"

"You got that right!"

"—but what you're not taking into consideration is that ours isn't the *only* kind of science. This is *occult* science. It's not from our world, it's from his.

192

Witchcraft and sorcery to you, but hard science to us. We think Eldred trance-channeled the instructions from Hell, then built the telly based on those specifications. And like so much potent magic ... a blood sacrifice is necessary." She looked right at him, eagerly, watching his expression.

"I'm not drinking any more of your blood," Farthing attested, "or anyone else's."

She sat up, turned, and face him directly. "You will if there's a gun to your cock. Jesus, Farthing! What have you got to lose? Do what they say, be a willing *part* of it like your uncle. Be rich, have everything you could ever want. For all that, all you gotta do is show 'em what they wanna see. Shit, most people would consider it an honor."

Farthing gaped. "Excuse me, an *honor?* To see torture and murder and mutilation? To see babies thrown to sharks and children napalmed?"

"Yes. An honor," she reiterated. "Nobody walking the earth has been able to see all those events, the most evil things to ever take place. Nobody but the Devil." Her brows rose. "And us."

It was impossible to juxtapose what she'd said with what he'd already witnessed. Something about her lewd pose dragged his eyes involuntarily down to her crotch. *For fuck's sake ...*

"Satan is just like God in a sense," she

continued. "He's omnipresent and all-knowing. He's everywhere and knows everything you're thinking and everything you've ever thought ..."

Well, in that case, he must know I'm thinking about your pussy ...

"... and I'm sure he'll throw you a bone before long."

"Throw me a *bone?*" he challenged. "What the hell does *that mean?*"

"Our benefactor can be kind and generous," Mal continued, "to those of his flock. He wants you on our side, Farthing. It's all for the proper cause. You'll realize that eventually." Her eyes darkened. "Sit up here on the bed with me."

"No," he said, and he couldn't have been more adamant.

She patted the mattress. "Come on. It don't look to me like you're very busy right now."

"No."

"Okay, if you don't want me to fuck your brains out again, then let's not beat around the bush. Let's go turn on the telly."

Farthing thought his face was shriveling up. "*Fuck* no."

She batted her eyelashes. "Pretty please?"

"No. I told you, I don't believe it. It's ridiculous. I don't believe in fuckin' occult *science.*"

"Why not?" she asked. She reached over and put her hand on Farthing's thigh.

"Stop it."

"Why not? Don't you believe that everything evolves?"

Farthing frowned hard. "What's that got to do with—"

"Science in our world has been evolving for thousands of years, right, love? So why wouldn't the science of Hell evolve at the same pace?" She squeezed his thigh and slipped her hand closer to his crotch.

Damn it. He was getting hard again. "Because there *is no Hell, and there's no Heaven or God or Devil or any of that shit. That's just stuff humans made up because they're creative and they want to explain why they're here and how the universe came to be. Every civilization has its own version of Heaven and Hell; it's all the same mythology.* Be good and you go to Heaven. Be bad, go to Hell."

Now she squeezed his crotch directly. "Okay, so if it's all rubbish, let's go do it anyway. Prove me wrong, show me how it's fake. Explain to me how that telly can do what it does." Eventually, she had his cock fully out of his pants and was teasing it with her hand. "And what if you're wrong?"

Farthing's awareness was going foggy with lust.

Was the room warmer? He remembered the fright he'd had previously when he thought he'd seen a dark figure in the hall. And he'd seen something like that outside too, hadn't he? But it turned out to be a post? And then there was the lone dark walker on the distant beach—walking toward him but seeming to make no progress. Farthing knew these things were illusions caused either by stress or drunkenness. But now, as Mal coddled his raw cock, he couldn't escape a similar notion: that a dark figure was in the room, just behind him. Seconds later, he felt a maddening impulse that he must look behind him to make sure no sinister man—or ghost—was in attendance. With great effort, he began to crane his neck—

"Turn your head this way," Mal said, then without warning, she emptied an eyedropper of some oily insipid liquid under his tongue. It was from that little bottle on the nightstand. "That should tune you up ..."

"What the fuck—" he gagged.

"It makes you harder than granite, love, and there's a little scopolamine in it too. Makes you more cooperative ..."

Distractions overwhelmed him; now Mal was on her knees, administering exemplary fellatio. The sensation had him on exotic pins and needles, he tensed up in the chair, was still trying to look behind him, but then Mal began to suck even more precisely, and the effort disintegrated. He was as hard as he'd ever been in his life.

Next, she was standing up, out of her panties again, and urging Farthing to stand. "Come on, love. If you want the rest, you come with me," and then, as if hypnotized, he was following her out of the bedroom, his cock still out, bobbing ludicrously.

For a split-second, the urge returned to look behind him, down the hall this time—

Is there really something there?

Describing it to himself would've been impossible, but at the very corner of his eye, he would swear he saw a tall thin man like a solid shadow, but when he fully turned his head, it wasn't there.

What was happening to him? Was he being manipulated against his will? If so, how? Whatever the case, he still felt dizzy with lust and confusion; his groin felt stuffed with the lewdest sensations. Next thing he knew, he was in the back room with the little ceiling light on, and he was sitting in the folding chair, facing the ancient television.

By now he felt undeniably drugged. His cock slid right into her when she plopped down in his lap, facing him. Her tongue pushed into his mouth and was roving around as she sucked on his breath. He could feel the hard points of her nipples poking him. Whatever the stuff was in the eyedropper bottle, it must be hallucinogenic as well as aphrodisic because it felt as though her tongue was swelling to the girth of a roll of cookie dough and sliding down to his stomach. When he was out of air, his body spasmed in the chair, and she held onto him tighter. It occurred to him that he was suffocating; he felt pin-pricks around his heart, in his lungs, moving up to his brain. It was only just before Farthing thought he'd die that she pulled her mouth off.

When he sat back, gasping, shuddering, almost mindless, she raised her arm, and with a knife she'd seemed to produce out of nowhere, she cut open her previous wound. "Do as I say," she said in a voice like crumbling rock. Her other hand yanked his head back by the hair, and she pressed her arm-wound tight against his open mouth. "Suck," she ordered. "Suck my blood out. Swallow it ..."

Overtly repulsed as he was ... Farthing sucked the wound. He sucked hard and swallowed the hot rusty fluid deep. His cock still buried in her, he was at the brink of orgasm, but it wouldn't quite release. After he'd sucked a few moments more, he saw the old TV screen come alight with, first, static fuzz, then—

On the screen, he saw a naked man and naked woman being stuffed into a thing like a large pinata, only it was made of bronze and it bore the shape of a bull. Men in leather armor finally got the unwilling captives into the bull, then closed and latched the metal door on top. A great wood fire was lit under the bull's belly, and there was a lapse of time until the nostrils of the bull began to emit steam. Later, the bull was rolled away from the fire, a bottom hatch was opened, and out fell the steamed, scarlet corpses.

One hundred haggard men stared forward; each had been lashed to a short fence in a long row, while a shirtless Japanese officer with a Rising Sun bandanna on his forehead intensely exerted himself as he moved down the line of captives, decapitating them each in one swipe with a Samurai sword. The idea was to kill one hundred Chinese men in as little time as possible. But then the scene bloomed into something else, a point of view detailing more Japanese soldiers forcing two Chinese families to rape each other; otherwise, the youngest child of each family would be skinned alive and throat-cut.

Russian soldiers exemplified themselves in a

Ukrainian apartment by gang-raping a woman and knifing her whilst forcing her children to watch. Then the children were protractedly water-boarded and drowned; several other soldiers were content to watch while masturbating. When the festivities were completed, the soldiers rummaged through the kitchen drawers for food.

And like a movie camera on fast-forward, another scene prolapsed before the visual perspective, this time a crowned woman sitting upon a gilt, cushioned chair, in the attitude of a queen. Bright white makeup covered her face but not quite effectively enough to hide the pocked remnants of smallpox. She wore a great bustled blue dress in the Tudor style, and she glittered with jewels and gold-trimmed buttons. Soldiers with breastplates and pikes stood about her, but it was *before her that the spectacle ensued: two adults and several children bound hand to foot, all lying, squirming, atop a pile of straw and* tinderwood. The queen smiled slightly when she nodded, and a soldier touched a pitch-torch to the tinder, and in a great *poof*, the pile went up in flames. Within the flames, the captives flipped and contorted; some nearly flipped themselves off the pyre, until the soldiers pushed them back in with their pikes.

And much like the queen, one of the Mughal

emperors of India leaned forward excitedly in his guarded rickshaw, gazing out into a stone-bordered field. There, staked to the ground with outstretched arms and legs, was a row of naked men and women; the woman on the end was very pregnant. When the Mughal was ready to behold the spectacle, he waved a hand, and out into the field came a tusked five-ton elephant, led by a trainer wearing a scarlet pagri and puffy shirt, carrying a stick like a conductor's wand.

The trainer waved the wand in a certain way, and the elephant approached the first captive and placed its huge foot across his waistline and groin, then the trainer jiggled the wand in a precise series of movements. The elephant's foot slowly stepped on the man's groin, pushing down, pushing down, the victim silently screaming, until his hips were crushed flat. The process was repeated on the next man, but this time the elephant's foot slowly crushed his ribcage, leaving him to convulse, almost comically wagging his head with his tongue out. Next lay the first woman, who screamed and shuddered in silence as the expertly trained creature, in very slow increments, lowered its foot to her face. The woman's back arched against her bonds, then went instantly slack as her skull was flattened, exploding gore like a red halo.

Variations of this process continued until the final woman—the pregnant woman—was reached. Here, the Mughal's interest sharpened to pinpoint acuity—he was literally sitting on the edge of his seat. Several spectators turned away, but not the Mughal, not his guards, and even the elephant, when commanded, seemed to hesitate, glancing momentarily at the trainer. But the wand zigged and zagged once more, and the elephant stomped down hard on the pregnant woman's distended belly, and the contents of her womb jettisoned an eruption of fetal gore at least twenty feet out from between her spread legs. The victim's remains continued to twitch and heave in place for several seconds. The Mughal raised his hands in delight, and—

—and next the viewpoint seemed to be dropped like a bomb before the face of whatever was watching, to show yet another pregnant woman's spread legs and bulging bare belly. This was very much a gynecological view: between the widely parted thighs, the hair-rimmed vulva could be seen, stretching, widening, opening, as a glistening bald head began to emerge, then the little shoulders, then the little arms, then a rubber-gloved hand took hold of the beautiful newborn babe, and a moment later, it was swaddled in a towel and handed to the white-gowned mother who'd just given birth to it. The new mother beamed in exuberance as she kissed and held her chubby creation. Then the point of view raised to the mother's face—

—Farthing awoke churning on the floor and yelling.

He couldn't see at first, as if the salvo of atrocities had blinded him. But he could feel. He felt a soft hand on his chest, rubbing, then felt the undisputable pulses of orgasm throbbing out of his cock, sperm vaulting into some unseen vagina. Eventually, whoever was sitting on him got off, and his just-spent erection began to go limp.

Whoever was touching his chest said, "That's a good boy. That's hittin' it like a porn star!"

Farthing's vision snapped back on. He was still on the floor, having obviously gotten out of the fold-down chair at some earlier time. The first thing his eyes registered was the image of Mal on her knees to his side, tweaking his nipples and grinning down. But then he looked up …

Someone had just climbed off him, and he saw that person, nude, walking out of the room.

It was Karen.

Mal chuckled. "Congratulations, Farthing. Now you're a bona fide fucker of children!"

"Fuck you!" he yelled when he realized the

implications. "I didn't know! I was unconscious!"

"A likely story," she chided.

"It was against my will!"

"Um-hmm," and then she showed him her cellphone screen. "You look pretty willing to me."

On the screen, he could see Karen sitting on his bare groin, moving up and down.

More blackmail, Farthing realized. *More coercion ...*

He noticed daylight framing the curtains. "I thought we were watching the TV. How long have I been lying on the floor? All night?"

Mal stood up and put her clothes back on; Farthing was getting sick of seeing her naked. "We watched the TV for a while," she said, "but when you couldn't take it anymore, you fell out of the chair and passed out. You kept dreaming, though, so I kept seeing it on the telly. Until the blood wore off."

Farthing pulled his pants up, exhausted, then buttoned his shirt. "I guess I have no choice but to believe all this now. It can't *all be hallucination.*"

"No, it can't, and it isn't. *None* of it is. And remember when I told you our benefactor would throw you a bone? That last one was it. That was your mother, wasn't it? Having a baby? And the baby was you."

Farthing gulped. "Yeah." *I got to watch my own birth ...*

Suddenly, she looked in awe. "You're so privileged. And I guess you don't even realize it."

"No, I don't."

"You will." She smiled lasciviously. "You're coming around."

I better not be ... "I still don't understand how this works," he said. "It's witchcraft? It's *magic?* Through some occult hocus pocus, the most horrific things ever witnessed by ... the devil ... are piped into that fucked up television, just so his worshipers can watch?"

"So they can *behold,* so they can *bear witness* to what *Lucifer* has witnessed," she corrected. "We're not exactly sure how it works. It's not the television that picks up the images, it's *you*—you're the receiver, due to your bloodline. Our benefactor transfers the vision to *you*—the things you see every night in your dreams, for example. And then it's *your* consciousness that projects those visions on the TV screen so that all of us can watch as well. Remember back in your parents' time, when you'd turn a radio on at first, it would take the electricity a few moments to warm up the tubes? Here, it's not electricity, it's blood—the blood of those who reject God. It's all a perfect example of occult science."

Farthing sat down on the chair and nearly sputtered. "So that's all this is? A satanic freakshow so you and your pals can see the worst things to ever happen in the world? Why? Why would you want to see shit like that?"

Mal came around and began to rub Farthing's shoulders. "When we're allowed to see what he has seen, that's the closest we'll ever come to being *like him. An eternal honor. And when we die, we'll be kings and queens in Hell.*"

Kings and queens in Hell, Farthing thought in an echo. *That's just fan-fuckin'-tastic ...*

Over time, Farthing supposed that he did indeed "come around." He stopped caring because caring had been reduced to futility. And it wasn't every night that the "group" came to the trailer to watch, just every now and then, special occasions: All Hallows, the Autumnal Equinox, some great warlock's death day. Mal had been pretty much tapped out from the start—you could only give so much blood in so much time before you became deficient—so the group bought blood from other, anonymous persons, persons who didn't ask questions. On such occasions, it wasn't just Saed,

Kirill, and Asenieth but a rotating retinue of very, very rich—and very, very evil—people from around the world: militaires, scientists, financiers, heads of state. As Farthing's psyche grew more cauterized to the atrocities on the TV and in his dreams, he took solace in his growing bank account—*huge* amounts of money wired into it. He even bought himself a McLaren and almost never drove it.

The basic ins and outs of his life scarcely changed; he simply continued being a boring retired senior citizen. He walked into town every so often, conversed cheerily with some neighbors, patronized the Mattshaw Pub at least twice a week enjoying small-talk with Bernice, and went for long walks on the beach in early evening. Sometimes, he thought he saw a lone distant figure in black moving toward him a mile or so off, but he could not be sure.

It was a great life—except when *they* came over. But he'd just bite the bullet and do what was expected of him.

Oh, and Mal and Karen kept coming over every day, and Farthing kept fucking them. Pervert? Child molester? That may well have been the case, but it wasn't like he had any choice. At any rate, before the first month was out, both girls were pregnant, and *more* money mysteriously appeared in Farthing's account.

Mal, of course, had had to take a long leave of absence from her job at the "shop," and she'd been content to live in the trailer with Farthing. Four months, five months, six—the more her belly enlarged, the lazier she became, until she'd reverted to the likes of most women from Farthing's past: a slouching, foul-mouthed free-loader. Intercourse was forbidden now; she could partake in no activity that might shake up the growing prize in her belly. However, she did bestow her oral expertise on Farthing most anytime he might want it. In fact, she even seemed heated for it and always swallowed his sperm without hesitation. Once she'd even said she felt thrilled to have "your cum in my belly," as if he were a rock star.

But to her and her group? He was far more than that. He was one who could make the television come on ...

Little Karen, on the other hand, was rarely seen again since the announcement of her successful pregnancy. It could only be presumed that Karen had been withdrawn from school for the time being. What could possibly explain a fourteen-year-old with a basketball-sized belly sitting in eighth-grade geometry class?

Walter, that gargantuan one-eyed thug, stopped by on occasion to check on things, or if not so much to check on things, to sodomize Mal when he had the fancy. No, intercourse was not allowed, but sodomy did not threaten the baby, so Walter had no qualms about having a go at Mal's "backdoor butler." All poor Mal would do was grin and bear it. Walter also liked to play cards and would force Mal to join him. "What's the bloody point?" she complained. "You always cheat." Farthing joined them one night but only for a single hand of poker. He quit when he noticed that the cards were adorned with photographs of masked men having sex with dead children.

And though the group only met periodically to watch the television—which, of course, required Farthing to chug a fair amount of blood—he was not spared the visual atrocity-show delivered by his dreams: the worst acts ever committed by humankind.

Einsatzgruppen and Sonderkommandos, before the war, would surreptitiously travel about Germany and round up the deformed, the disabled, retardates, elderly invalids, and mental patients by the thousands—anyone determined to be a liability to the Reich. Then they'd be quietly trucked off to "new care facilities," but alas, what really happened was that they were exterminated *en masse* and either buried in woodland trenches or cremated. Once the war had started, these paramilitary members were specifically separated into brigades whose missions were to go from village to village and town to town in eastern Poland, the Ukraine, and Belarus and murder all civilians, including women and children, so that the Reich's self-proclaimed *Lebensraum,* or living space, would not be tainted by Slavic genes. Einsatzgruppen troops, in fact, were at liberty to rape women and children as they saw fit, in order to dispel battlefield anxiety.

More of Farthing's nightmares included much of the procedures of Imperial Japan's Manshu Detachment Unit 731, which set up research facilities in northeast China, where all manner of lethal experiments were conducted against captives, particularly babies, children, and pregnant women. These experiments included forced infections, chemical agent applications, and barometric pressure fluctuations. Pregnant women were vivisected alive and filmed; many others were transfused with animal blood or simply over-filled with human blood to see what happened, subjected to controlled amputations, systematically exsanguinated, frozen or boiled at indexed temperatures, surgically flensed to determine how long they could live without skin. Brain transplants were attempted, or brain "plugs" were removed from one live subject and implanted into the live brain of another. Research from the facility was also principal in the development of aerosolized chemical and biological materials that were tested actively on more remote Chinese towns. After the war, the United States Office of Strategic Services offered amnesty to any Japanese medical personnel who agreed to report the results of their experiments, and cash payments were offered for written and photographic research records.

Multinational Wagner Group mercenaries, armed by Russia, were paid to fight "rebels" who opposed the puppet government in the Central African Republic. These fine soldiers were deployed once to the town of Létélé and ordered to make examples of the rebels; their favorite procedure was to disembowel women and children alive and leave their eviscerated bodies in the streets for all to see. In no long time, however, hyenas in the surrounding jungle smelled the blood and invaded the area, eating every human being they could find, alive or dead, including some of the Wagner personnel.

Illinois serial-killer and pervert John Wayne

Gacy liked to perform fellatio on his handcuffed victims and then put make-shift tourniquets on their necks. He would insert a pen beneath the rope and use it in a relief-valve-type process, tightening and loosening, tightening and loosening, over and over again, always staring directly into the victim's eyes. John wanted his pudgy, insane face to be the last image to register in the victim's brain when he ceased to exist. Then John would sodomize the dead body and bury it in a crawlspace in his basement. Eventually, twenty-six bodies were buried there.

Another famed serial-killer, California's Edmund Kemper, whenever he had an argument with his overbearing mother, would pick up attractive hitchhikers, kill them, dismember them and cut off their heads, and then have sex with the heads via an act called *irrumatio*. There was one head he was particularly fond of having sex with, and he kept it accessible for several days. Eventually, he murdered his belligerent mother and had sex with her severed head too.

It was images such as these that Farthing was forced to see either on the old television or in his nightly dreams, and over time, he began to feel as though his very *soul* were being marinated in chuckling, undiluted evil. His self-concept was changing, *spoiling,* and he didn't care. Over time, a part of him began to feel impressed, even honored—as Mal had said—to witness the worst things ever perpetuated by mankind.

Sometimes he even smiled as he watched the untold atrocities.

By now, he knew that it was all true; he knew that these were indeed visions beheld by the Devil, which meant that he *believed* in the Devil, and if he believed in the Devil, then he subsequently *must* believe in God. Hence, the choice of to whom to pledge his faith was before him: God or the Devil?

Farthing chose the latter.

Months later, into winter, when Mal and Karen were the better part of seven months pregnant, Farthing thought more intricately on what that really meant.

It meant that his uncle's bloodline would carry on, and with it, the ability to continue operating the television, to purvey the visions of Satan to his most faithful clan. But of course, this also meant that the clan would no longer have any reason to keep Farthing alive. He'd be replaced by one of the babies he'd sired, and they would probably use Farthing's blood for the earliest activations, and, no doubt, they'd use *all of it, till he was bone-dry, and then get rid of his body. One of the children would pick up the task from there.*

Still, that child, or both of them, would have to be raised and properly indoctrinated by Saed and his "Group," and this would likely take *years,* wouldn't it? So Farthing reasoned that until then, he would continue to be indispensable to the clan. *Years,* he thought with some satisfaction. His life, and all its new-found diabolical trimmings, wasn't over just yet.

Therefore, Farthing reasoned that he'd have as much fun as he could, and most of that fun involved the admission of his erection into Mal's mouth. Once, after she'd swallowed it all, he'd observed, "You must be sick to death of sucking my old cock," but she beamed in her response, "It's my job to keep you happy, and I love my job. It's a privilege!"

The transformation from what he'd been to what he was now couldn't have been more shocking. Unassuming and drab nice guy one day and Satanic preceptor the next. For his abilities, he was being treated like a king. Anything he wanted, they would give him, but in truth, all he wanted was to revel in his dreams or watch the horror on the television. He'd even, to his eternal shame, cum in *Karen's mouth a few times, or spewed on her bulbous stomach, and his reaction was only this: I just came on a pregnant fourteen-year-old's stomach. Big fuckin' deal ...*

They even said he could travel anywhere he wanted, as long as Walter went with him and he wasn't gone for more than a few weeks. But the desire strangely wasn't there. All that served his interests now were the monstrous images his ancestry allowed him to see.

One clear winter night, Farthing sat outside in the fenced-in rear-yard. He drank beer and gazed up at the moon and the spill of stars, shadowed by the copper globe that he understood contained Eldred's ashes. Some tropish statuary stood amongst the clumps of shrubbery and the empty bird bath: dead-eyed cherubs and prayerful angels with broken off faces. Of course, there remained several black posts which supported empty flower pots, and now as he nursed his ale, he stared hard at one such post, and he recalled one of his first nights at the trailer: he'd been convinced that a slender, dark-dressed man was standing there, staring back, but when he blinked out of the mirage, he found himself staring at nothing more than the black post.

When such a mirage returned now, he was

prepared to attribute it to errant drunkenness. Farthing sat in a patio chair and did indeed identify a figure standing before him, the same dark, slender thing that seemed to move ever-so-minutely. It was like when one stared at something for so long, and not blinking at all, that *something* became something *else.* Farthing addressed the figure lackadaisically, with no fear, and even smiled.

"Is that you, Uncle Eldred?" he ventured. "Your ghost? Are you really there?" Farthing squinted harder. "Yes, I really think it *is* you …" Did the figure then actually point at him? He couldn't be sure in the darkness. "So, you're the honcho here, you're the kingpin, is that right? This whole big Satanic shebang is being conducted by you …" Farthing began to feel a buzzing sensation all about his body when, this time, the figure held up its black hands. Its left hand showed five fingers, and its right hand showed one. Then the gesture was repeated twice more. Farthing had to chuckle to himself. "Six-six-six? Not very original, Uncle Eldred." But now the figure was pointing down to the area of cement space that existed between Farthing's feet.

He set down his beer and leaned over, staring at that same area. The white of the cement looked gray in the moon-tinted darkness, and then his brow furrowed when he saw, or *thought he saw, a jet-black spot on the cement, yes, a black spot the size of a quarter or perhaps a half-dollar.*

Something forced him to disregard all impulses except to continue to stare at the black spot, and as he did so, his vision began to warp, until it became plain to him that the spot was no spot at all but a hole, a *jet-black* hole, and then he grew overwhelmed by an intractable curiosity and a misery of anxiety, and suddenly there was nothing more important than making sure that the spot was really a hole.

So he leaned over harder and put his finger into the hole past the first two joints, but he withdrew his finger fast as he might, for a considerable *heat wafted up from the hole. And next he closed one eye and stared, stared down hard into the unfathomable hole*, and soon his vision began to sink deeper, deeper and down into the seemingly incalculable depths of the impossible aperture.

How deep *was* the hole, and what purpose did it serve? Where did it stop?

Then he heard a scrabbling sound, and with that came a certainty that some macabre terror threatened to issue itself from the hole, and the harder and harder he stared, movement presented itself, *upward* movement, and as Farthing's breath caught in his chest and he began to smell noxious smoke, he saw that the movement was comprised of a *figure* with a face, a *human* face, and a *charred* one at that. Up, up, and up it climbed, faster and faster, as if its goal were not to escape its fiery confines but to reach out and grab on to the oblivious, interloping head that leaned over the hole. When the appalling eidolon seemed about to emerge, Farthing fell forward, smacked his head on the cement, and fell immediately into unconsciousness, but not before he took note of the menacing figure's face. It was Farthing's own.

Farthing awoke the next day, sometime in the afternoon, in bed and with a raging headache. When his vision sharpened, he was shocked to notice a half dozen people looking down on him, their faces all imprinted with looks of deep concern. There was Saed, Kirill, Asenieth, and Mal, plus another well-dressed elderly gentleman Farthing didn't know.

"There he is!" announced Saed. "Back among us at last."

"That's quite a spill you took last night," Mal suggested. "We found you sprawled out flat on the cement, out cold and bleeding. But the doctor's set you back to rights."

"Mr. Farthing," said the unknown man. "I'm Dr. Lawrence. You friends sent for me at once, and I had you transported to the hospital where, I'm happy to inform you, we found that your head-wound is minor and you've not suffered any manner of fracture. I'm afraid you'll be groggy for a day or two—you see, you've suffered a slight concussion. But I think I can safely say you're out of the woods. Just take it easy next few days, and call me if anything changes." And with that, the doctor put away his stethoscope, grabbed his bag, and left.

"You gave us all quite a scare," Asenieth said. "You must be very careful."

"What caused you to fall?" Kirill asked pointedly.

"I," Farthing began, and then he thought back to the entire thing. What could he tell them? *A hole to Hell formed in the patio ...* "I'm ashamed to say," he said, "that I was a wee bit drunk, and I must've tripped. I'm terribly sorry to have caused so much trouble."

"No matter, that," Saed replied, then chuckled, "Just—please—be more careful in the future!"

Mal, fully dressed now and stomach bulging

away, squeezed his hand. "Like the doctor just say, get plenty of rest. I'll be out here if you need anything, love."

"Thank you."

He did begin to feel better soon, so he took a shower and dressed. The throbbing beneath the bandage on his forehead had abated. In the living room, only Mal sat, sidled over on the couch asleep, her fingers laced over the belly that contained Farthing's child. There was no sign of Walter.

With nothing better to do, he went out the front door and walked around to the rear of the trailer, re-facing the posts, the statues, and the shrubbery he remembered from last night. And there stood the chair that he'd sat down in when he fell over; in fact, there was a small smudge of blood at the place where he'd scraped his head. This was the first time he'd noticed that the back patio area was not covered by poured cement but instead by square cement tiles.

Why the notion occurred to him, he couldn't guess, but a moment later, he was rooting around in the cobweb-festooned garden shed, which he hadn't opened since he'd moved here. A gas-powered weed-trimmer and canister of fuel, rakes, hoes, a shovel, and various tools were the most obvious contents. He found an old paint-scraper and a screwdriver, and was next sitting right back in the patio chair from last night. The gap between the cement tiles was just wide enough to admit the edge of the paint-scraper, and this he wedged back and forth with all his senior-citizen might until a gap had widened large enough to stick the screwdriver in. From there, prying the tile up was the work of a minute or two.

He lifted the tile away and was now looking down at something that had deliberately been secreted beneath: a green metal combination safe.

Somebody buried a fuckin' floor-safe in here! he realized.

Too many speculations were percolating in his head now. Had Eldred put this here, and meant to conceal it from the group? Or had the group put it here? He had to find out, but now wasn't the time—it was broad daylight and anyone might see him.

At least the safe's presence provided a tidbit of intrigue. He instantly replaced the tile, an almost automatic action. If this indeed were a secret safe deposited by Saed and company, he had to know why. And if the safe contained things that Eldred had wished to conceal from the entire group … well, that propelled a curious tangent, didn't it? Most of all, however …

I gotta find out what's inside, he thought.

He moved the chair away from the tile—as if *that* would deflect suspicion that he'd been prying into business that was not his own!—and stashed the screwdriver and scraper in a bush, then moseyed around the lot to seem nonchalant. Brief glances at the windows told him that no one was spying on him, and then he felt a bit ludicrous letting his paranoia go that far.

While walking around the front, he espied the Cat Lady (who was followed, as always, by a queue of cats). "Hi, how are you today?" Farthing attempted a greeting, but she only looked over at him, grinned, then continued on her way.

Great talking to you too, bitch. I've seen you naked, by the way.

Without forethought then, he walked into town and, as it were, passed a shop whose glass window read HAWBERK & SONS - LICENSED LOCKSMITHS, which reminded him again of the combination safe hidden beneath his patio tile. *Maybe I'll be calling on Mr. Hawberk soon,* he thought. Either that or he'd have to look around and see if Uncle Eldred might have jotted down the combination somewhere—if indeed it had been Eldred who'd planted the safe. It seemed unlikely that a man in his nineties would be able to commit something like that to memory—at least, Farthing couldn't: all his passwords were scribbled on index cards taped under his desk. Still, Farthing felt a nearly implacable desire to find out what was in that safe …

Next thing he knew, the cowbell was ringing and in he walked to the Mattshaw Pub. No conscious impulse—except perhaps alcoholism—had steered him here.

"Ah, my favorite Yank, back again," Bernice greeted and had a beer poured for him without asking. "So what happened to you? Some bird's angry husband get the best of ya?"

He touched the fat bandage on his forehead. "Nothing so interesting as that. I got drunk last night and fell over."

"Well, then, this here'll put you on proper footing," she said and slid the beer to him. "Haven't seen you in a while. Been away?"

No, I've been busy getting sucked into a Satanic cult and knocking up two girls, one of whom is fourteen. "Just puttering around the new place."

"Liking it, are ya?"

"Yes, I do," he lied. "Everyone is so nice, and the park is so quiet. In America, I wasn't used to that. Where I used to live, a night wouldn't go by that I didn't hear gunshots and sirens."

Bernice crossed her arms beneath her copious bosom. "That's because we ain't all savage-like 'ere in jolly ole England. Had a couple thousand years more than you to get civilized."

The theorem sounded like a credible one. "Yorkshire Ripper notwithstanding, I agree with you."

A few other customers came in, which required Bernice's temporary departure. Sitting by himself in a bar suited him well; he was not responsible for entertaining someone else or conducting himself any special way. *Just nice and quiet, he thought. He was sick of shifty people coming and going at the trailer, he was sick of Saed's people and their "blackmail." He was even getting sick of Mal and her propensity of walking around naked with her distended* stomach sticking out and her milk-enlarged breasts. The only thing he *wasn't* sick of was—

My God …

—the abominable nightmares he saw every night and the even-worse visions that sunk into his head when the "group" came over. Anyone else would be permanently nauseated, but not Farthing.

Why?

He actually found that he *looked forward* to the appalling visions. How could anyone look forward to seeing such things? Even as he quietly considered the question, a roulette-wheel of images spun round his mind's eyes: corpse-piles set aflame in Africa, Belsen SS catching babies on bayonets, Roman soldiers raping Carthaginian women in the dirt. Farthing could only sit there and stare back into the visual chasm as his cock grew insufferably hard.

That's the only answer. I'm becoming like them — like Saed and Kirill and the rest of those Satanic psychos. Farthing gulped. *I'm becoming evil …*

He nearly yelped when someone pulled up the stool beside him, and then a hand settled on his thigh. It was Mal.

"Should'a known I'd find ya here," she said, none too pleased. "Thanks for invitin' me. You sure know how ta make a girl feel wanted."

Shit … He just wanted to sit by himself. "I'm not going to invite a pregnant woman to a bar, for God's sake. It's not like you can drink anything."

She'd taken to wearing stretch skirts now, due to her ballooning stomach. And pulled down over that was a black Eddie & the Hotrods t-shirt with a hangman's noose on it. Her milk-filled breasts were now twice as large as when he'd met her, with nipples sticking out like baby pacifiers. "I'm tickled you're so concerned for my well-being."

She lewdly squeezed his thigh, then jerked her hand closer to his crotch.

Bernice came over, a sly smile on her face.

"Bernice, this is Mal, Mal this is Bernice," Farthing sloppily introduced.

Mal nodded, and Bernice said, shooting a quick glance to Mal's stomach, "Pleased to meet ya, darlin'. What'll it be?"

"An OJ, please."

When Bernice disappeared for the orange juice, Mal's hand went straight to Farthing's crotch and squeezed. "So what the shit're you doin' snufflin' up that old bint's arse?"

Farthing pulled her hand off and glared. "I'm having a beer. What are *you* doing here?"

She put her hand right back on his crotch, rubbing this time. "Just makin' sure you're okay. I told ya, it's my job to keep you happy—"

"I'm perfectly happy *without* your hand on my junk!" he whispered.

"Sure don't feel like it here," she whispered back, grinning. "Sure feels like there's *something hard in there that might need* tendin' too."

He pulled her hand off again.

"I'll wank this right here'n now under the bartop, and that big-tit-bitch won't care. Shit, I'll bet that water buffalo's jerked off hundreds of blokes here for a couple quid each …"

"You shouldn't even be out!" he snapped back, then glanced at the bulbous belly. "Your stomach looks like an overcooked Jiffy Pop—"

Mal smirked. "A *what?*"

"You look like you could drop any minute. Do you really want to do that in a *bar?*"

She laughed just as Bernice reappeared and set down the orange juice, cocked a brow at Farthing, then walked away again. "*Relax,* love! I ain't due for another month. And don't change the subject. Next time you fancy a bit of a walk, you take me with ya. It's safer."

Farthing winced. "Safer? *Why?*"

"Well, you're no spring chicken, right? You could get confused 'n' get yourself lost. You could fall down 'n' break your bloody hip—"

"Fuck you," he muttered. "I'm not *that old. Yet.*"

"We should leave this fuckin' outhouse 'n' go back to the trailer. So's I can take care 'a you proper-like."

"No. I'm enjoying my beer, or trying to." He swallowed a gulp, then grimaced at a thought. "So when's your group meet again?"

"It ain't *my* group, love. Those twisted knob-ends are *your* group. I'm just the hired help."

"The Satanic baby factory, you mean …"

Mal chuckled.

"So answer the question," Farthing went on. "When do I have to turn that goddamn TV on again?"

"The Solstice," she said. "You know, only on the special days."

Farthing rolled his eyes. "Great. When's the fuckin' *Solstice* then?"

"Tomorrow …"

Farthing slouched. *Fuck. So soon?* But it only felt like *half* a reaction. One part of him dreaded it, the other part seemed excited. *Yeah. Some weird shit's happening to me.* He checked to make sure Bernice was out of earshot. "So where are they getting the blood now? They can't use any more of yours, not with that bun in the oven."

"Oh, no, a preggered chick's blood is super, it's even better. But they don't take it from me anymore, nor Karen neither. The babies need ours. They just go out of town a bit and buy it from homeless rummies and the like."

Homeless rummies, Farthing repeated. *Fantastic. And I have to drink it …*

"And I guess it's goin' on three-quarters of a year you been doing it. I'm surprised you haven't started slipping."

Farthing looked at her, annoyed. "*Slipping?*

228

What the hell are you talking about now?"

"After you do it enough times, and your brain gets used to it, and your spirit too. Then you'll start to …" but then her words trailed off and she made a smug smile. "No. Best you wait. You'll know it when it happens. Eldred said slipping was his favorite part."

Anger flashed; Farthing grabbed her arm and was surprised by how hard he squeezed it. "No. Tell me now. What do you mean by slipping?"

She looked at his hand gripping her. "That *hurts*, Farthing. I didn't think roughin' birds up was your style."

He released her arm, but his anger flared harder. "What's slipping?"

She let out a deep breath. "It was Eldred who told me all about it," she began, "and giddy as a schoolboy, he was when tellin' me. After your psyche gets attuned to things—"

"*Attuned?*"

"Yeah, love. Your psyche, your spirit, your soul—whatever you wanna call it. Whenever that gets used to what ya dream and what ya see on the telly … then you start ta kind of *slip into it*—"

Farthing, ever more impatient, ground his teeth. "Slip into *what?*"

She leaned over, whispering more lightly.

"Whatever it be you're dreamin' or watchin' on the screen. Eldred say it gets so you're not really *watchin' the stuff anymore, but you're doing it, doin' it with your own two hands.*"

Farthing seemed to hold his breath, thinking about that. *Not watching. Doing.* What would that be like? Would he even be able to stomach it?

"Eldred told me, first time it happened to him, he were watchin' on the telly some evil bloke dropping some women and kids into a well-hole, and then he 'n' some other fellas started dropping manhole covers on top of 'em, and before the vision was over, it was *Eldred himself helping toss in them manhole covers. Another time, he said, he was watching inquisitors or some such*—in Spain, he thought—jabberin' in front of three naked witches tied to stakes, and next thing he knew, Eldred was *in* the vision, and it was he himself putting the torch down to the kindling and settin' fire to them three women. Said he could see their skin blacken right afore him, could hear 'em poppin' and cracklin', and he said he could feel the heat on his face watchin' them women twitch ..."

Farthing tried to picture that and compare it against all the evil, horrid visions he'd seen over these past months. Nausea started to rise but then went back down again, and he could feel his erection pulsing in his pants. Then he looked down at her stretched belly, then at her bare legs, then at her nipples sticking out under the t-shirt.

"Likin' whatcha see?" Mal coyly asked.

He left a hefty overpayment on the bartop. "Let's get out of here. Your body's fuckin' killing me."

"Oh, is it now! Finally startin' to appreciate me, are you?"

In a few beats of his heart, he was no longer himself. He just wanted to fuck her, and he didn't want to putter around. He said a haphazard goodbye to Bernice, grabbed Mal's hand, and practically pulled her off the stool.

"What's with you all of a sudden?" she asked, amused.

He grimaced when the daylight hit him in the face, but then that same daylight seemed to darken, as though some clouds passed over.

He looked up; there were no clouds.

The sudden darkening must be in his mind.

"In here for a minute," he said and pulled her into a narrow alley. He grabbed her hand and forced it down his pants. Then he pressed her against a brick wall next to some stacks of delivery crates and began to knead her breasts; she must've liked it because she took in a deep breath and rose on her tiptoes. Then she did it again when he slipped one hand up her skirt—it was no surprise she was pantiless—and began to finger her. Her clitoris felt hard as a jellybean. His free hand came off her breast and grabbed her throat, squeezing. "Feel up my cock, for shit's sake. You're not exactly a novice."

Semi-shocked, she did as ordered, fondling his balls, squeezing his erection until wet dots appeared on his pants. She was staring at him now in a vicious lust.

One hand squeezed her breast; it began to leak milk into her black shirt. He squeezed harder, till she winced, and then his other hand re-found her throat and squeezed so hard her face began to pinken. The effort made him madly hard. *Limey cunt,* he thought. *I should choke her out. Fuck it. Why not? Just kill her and put her out with the rest of the trash ...*

Finally, she reacted and forced his hand off her throat. "What the fuck's wrong with you, Farthing? I don't mind things a little rough, but—fuck!—you should see your face! You look like you wanna fuckin' *kill* me."

Do I? He ignored her and continued fingering her. One finger, two, then three. "I'm gonna fist you. See if that doesn't tamp down your sass—"

"Noo!" she squealed in a whisper. "You could break my water! You'll fuck up the kid—"

"I could shit care less about the kid," he said, and put in a fourth finger. "I hope it's born with flippers. Probably will be, from all the drugs *you've* taken."

Her eyes were daggers now, sinking into his own. "What the *fuck* is WRONG with you?"

His hand squirmed just outside of the slick slot. Was he really going to put his entire fist in her?

She began to lurch against him. "Farthing, if I lose this baby, those people will fuckin' *kill me!*"

"That's not my problem," he grunted, but he called his own bluff and took his hand away, only to push her down on her knees. "You said your job's to make me happy? Well, make me happy," and he took his erection out and grabbed a handful of her multicolored hair. "Suck that. Get it good and wet." He pushed it into her mouth, began to hump her face right there with her big stomach sticking out and the back of her head against the bricks. He wanted to cum right down her throat— because that's all her throat really was: a drain for errant seed; and that's all *she* was: a container for his *use*. He was about to push his cock all the way to the back of her throat and choke her but reneged at the last second. *The cunt would probably bite me, then I'd REALLY have to kill her …*

She looked winded and cross-eyed when he pulled her back up. Were there actually tears in her eyes? He hoped so.

"For pity's sake!" she said. "It's broad daylight! Someone's gonna see!"

"Does it look like I care?" He pushed her shirt up, put a nipple in his mouth, and just sucked. Sweet, hot milk sprayed against his tongue. Then he spun her around so fast, she squealed; he pushed her cheek and stomach against the brick. That compulsion kept flaring back: to choke her hard, to wring her fucking neck, and make that baby drop. Is that what would happen? If the bitch died, would the baby just fall out? Would the dead womb eject it?

He reached both hands around her stomach and squeezed hard. He could feel something in there, something like lumps, something moving.

Now Mal sounded terrified. "Farthing, you're being too rough—"

In response, he buffeted the side of her bulging stomach with his fist.

"You're insane! Stop it!"

"Every time you say something, I'll hit that big belly harder," and then he hit it again.

Hearing her sobs only hardened his cock even

more. He crooked his head over, let a large glob of spit fall directly from his mouth into her ass crack, pushed her buttocks open, and sunk his erection unhesitantly into her anus.

Mal tensed all up, still sobbing. "At least have the decency to warn a girl first, you prick ..."

Decency doesn't seem to be on the menu today, he thought. The sensation was delectable, almost electric: her rectal canal spasming around his cock as it banged in and out. "That's it," he muttered, "that's it, you cunt, you fuckin' cum-dump." She squealed again at another hard twist of her hair, and next he was cringing, his cock emptying its orgasm deep into her bowels. Yeah, and that smug little Karen bitch'll be next. I'll bust that fourteen-year-old pussy UP and make the kid retarded. I'll fuck her so hard, the kid'll think it's in a washer machine. Only two raw emotions filled every fiber of Farthing's being now: lust and hatred. He felt *glowing* with it.

When the last spurt of semen made its exit, Farthing pulled his cock out and shoved Mal aside; she stumbled and fell over but Farthing didn't care. He pulled his pants back up, was about to refasten his belt, but caught himself looking down at her, and all that was in his head was a blind sick rage. He could see himself kicking her in the head, kicking her in the belly, stomping her. Next thing he knew he was reaching for his cock again. He wanted to *piss* on her too, piss all over her, then yank her head back and piss more in her mouth— really finish off her day on a good note ... but then, just like a pencil being broken in half, he snapped out of it, and that dark tint in the sky brightened. Everything that he'd just done flooded back into his head, to his horror.

What have I done? Holy shit! I just raped her!

He couldn't have rushed over fast enough to help her back to her feet. She was wobbly and still teary eyed.

"Mal, holy shit! I'm sorry! Here, let me help you—"

She gagged, blindly swinging her fists at him. "God damn you, you sick shit ..." She pulled her skirt up to squint at her pubis, checking for blood. "If I lose this kid, I swear I'll kill you before they can kill me ..."

"I'm sorry," he kept pathetically repeating. "I'm sorry." And then he grabbed her and hugged her.

She stiffened up at first, then relaxed. "I guess that's what I get for agreein' to do this shit for those fuckers."

Farthing stroked her cheek. "I'm sorry, Mal. I-I don't know what came over me."

"I do," she said.

236

Mal pretty much collapsed on the bed when they got back to the trailer, curled up into as much of a fetal position as her physique would permit. She was fast asleep.

Fuckin'-A ... Farthing was still shocked at himself, now more than ever as he stared down at her, wide-eyed.

He tried to wonder what life was like for her, and he didn't like the thoughts that returned. *Shitty family life—if she even HAD an intact family, shitty childhood, exploitation and sexual abuse from an early age.* The same old story for so many. No dreams of the future. Nothing to ever be happy about. Just johns and dirty old men and God knew what else.

And then along comes me, beating the shit out of her, and FUCKING the shit out of her. Just what she needs, especially when she's eight months pregnant. How the hell could I do that to her?

He supposed he knew but just hadn't quite made the self-acknowledgment. *This fuckin' trailer, that fuckin' TV, and Saed and his group of psychos.* It was insinuating itself into Farthing, seeping into his blood and his psyche. *All thanks to my FUCKIN' Uncle Eldred ...*

A devil-worshiper ...

With Mal dead asleep and no one else in the house, Farthing thought it safe to go out to the backyard. There was still the matter of that safe hidden under the patio tile.

So back Farthing went to the area where the globe was and the garden. The lawn chair remained where he'd left it, and when he sat down, he looked about and listened for signs of others. Finding none, he bent over, retrieved the paint scraper and screwdriver, and had the cement tile prized out in only moments. He tried the safe handle, but of course, it wouldn't open, *Fuck. What did I expect?* He dialed in the trailer's street address on the combination knob, then Eldred's birthday, and—nothing. Then a notion slammed into his head, as if by an exterior force. *Wait a min—*

He recalled last night's mirage, or alcohol-induced hallucination. *Yes ...* The black figure standing before his drunken eyes and how it seemed to have made hand gestures: one hand opened showing all five fingers, the other hand closed, save for a single figure, six black fingers showing in all. Then the gesture was repeated twice more.

No, Farthing thought, frowning. That's too easy, but he saw no harm in giving it a try.

He touched the safe's knob, dialed in six-six-six,

then turned the handle—

click

No fucking way! The safe opened.

He wasn't quite sure what he expected: a hand of glory, voodoo dolls, vials of occult potions? But nothing of the sort returned his cruxed gaze. The only thing that occupied the safe was a large pistol—an old revolver—and a box of ammunition whose faded label read HORNADY .455 WEBLEY.

What the fuck? Why hide a gun out here?

Actually, though, there might be a very sound reason. If Uncle Eldred had been as much under the control of the group as Farthing was, then a gun might have come in handy in case they turned on him. He'd secured it out here to reduce the chance of Walter or Saed or someone finding it. But as Farthing reflected further on the possibility, he heard the sound of a car door closing out front, and it could only be from his driveway.

Goddamn it …

He scrambled to put the gun and bullets back in the safe, close it, and re-cover the hole. Then he nonchalantly ambled about the garden area with the sprinkler can. *Look normal,* he told himself.

He expected someone to come outside to see what he was up to, but that didn't happen. Now, voices were heard from the living room area—

Saed and company, no doubt. But then he heard Mal's voice from the bedroom, objecting, "Give a girl a break, will ya! I've 'ad a bad day!" "You'll know what a bad day really is if you don't have my John Thomas in your yap in two seconds," came Walter's voice.

The curtains over the French doors had just enough of a gap for Farthing to peek in, and there was Walter, the eye-patched giant, with his pants down and an overly large erection pushing against Mal's pressed lips. She shook her head, wasn't going for it, until—

CRACK!

—Walter laid an open hand across her face so hard it sounded like a low-caliber pistol shot. Mal fell back on the bed, hands to face, and then she squealed when Walter yanked her t-shirt up, bent over, and bit hard into her nipple. She squirmed as if electrified.

"I'll bite it off," he said calmly, "I swear. Now, are you gonna suck this cock or not?"

"Yes, yes!" she yelled.

"Good. Then do it. Do what you were put on Earth for, ya sauce-box, or I'll *really* give ya somethin' to throw a wobbly over—"

Farthing could only watch through the gap for a few seconds as Mal did as commanded. Walter vised her head with both hands and fucked her face, not caring when she gagged. All the while, Farthing mused, *Yeah, that's one big fucker I'd LOVE to kill,* and he could, couldn't he? He could open that safe back up, grab the gun, and blow Walter's head off right in the middle of his blowjob. *How cool. Then I'd kill the rest of those sick fucks in the living room, use their brains to make some American modern art …*

But he did nothing of the sort. He averted his eyes from the gap and heard Walter muttering, "That's a good little bitch. Swallow it all; just like porridge, ain't it? Gotta keep that baby well-fed …"

Poor Mal, Farthing thought, depressed. First, she gets her ass kicked by me, and now, THAT big piece of British shit …

He walked back around to the front door, passing a sangria-red Rolls Royce. All heads looked up cheerily when he entered. Saed sat at one end of the couch, flipping through the old photo album of Eldred's nude Polaroids, Asenieth, in a sage-gray dress, next to him, and Kirill was at the kitchen counter making coffee. His borscht- and caviar-filled belly was pushing out like a sandbag against a thousand-dollar Versace silk shirt.

"Ah, Mr. Farthing!" Saed greeted. "So nice to

see you. I hope your minor head wound hasn't been too troubling."

"I'm too drunk to feel it much," he said, then brushed past Kirill and got a beer out of the fridge.

Saed chuckled while Asenieth glared right at Farthing's face, then his crotch through narrowed eyes and a vulturine grin. "Sit, sit, please," Saed said. "We must talk."

Farthing sat down in the armchair. From this angle, he could see Asenieth's bare pubis because she had just uncrossed her legs, the folds of the vulva very apparent. *Sharon Stone you ain't,* he thought. *Is that a pussy or a Turkish delicatessen?*

"What we need to make you aware of," Saed began, "are the important events approaching with the season."

"I gotta feeling you're not talking about Christmas," Farthing said.

"No, Mr. Farthing, not Christmas but something much older, older than Bethlehem and Babylon, older than Knossos, older than human history. And one common denominator for all this time immemorial is the winter solstice. We're told that it was a great thanksgiving for the end of the sun's wane, marking a return to light. But others, for ten thousand years or more, have celebrated the winter solstice as the darkest day of the year, the day when the least amount of sunlight falls upon the earth." Saed smiled at Farthing. "It's a very *powerful* time, Mr. Farthing, especially to our ilk. It's a time when our benefactor bestows his greatest blessings, a time when the supremely privileged — yourself, for example—become conduits of the greatest magnitude."

Farthing's lips pursed. "I get it. The winter solstice is party time for you and your crew, and I'm gonna have to turn on the TV—so everyone can get their jollies."

Saed rolled his eyes. "I suppose that's as good a way of putting it as any. But I'd think that after all this time of acclimation, you'd be a bit more enthusiastic. Whether you like it or not, you *are* one of us now, and I think you may be starting to enjoy the visions far more than you're letting on."

Farthing's cock still tingled in his pants. "Maybe I am, but so what? I know you've got me under your thumb, I'll do the shit you want me to do, and I know I don't have a choice. So there's not much to talk about really. Just tell me what time tomorrow to be ready."

Saed gave a satisfactory nod. "Dusk."

"Got it." Farthing rose, then went back outside—he supposed to spend the rest of the day drinking.

Many beers later, he dragged himself to bed.

He flopped down right next to Mal. She was murmuring in some somnambulistic turmoil. When he opened his eyes to stare at the dark, he thought he detected movement at the farthest fringes of his vision, and when he closed them, he saw a background of some dark color he couldn't describe, but eventually, letters formed: squiggles and slashes, warped geometric shapes, and the tiniest rune-like sigils. Some wholly unconscious urge made him press his groin against Mal's ass, which his cock had already marauded once today. He yanked the seat of Mal's skirt up, baring her buttocks. His hardness returned at once, but there was no lust in it, only revulsion at himself and a nausea like motion-sickness. In fact, the idea of sodomizing her again made him feel utterly suicidal, for he knew these desires did not come from him; they came from somewhere—or someone—else. He was being manipulated and he knew it. His erection raged again, he got it out, was about to spit on it and stick it back in Mal's ass, but bit his lip till he bled and masturbated instead, spewing all over her buttocks and the backs of her thighs. His orgasm felt cringingly potent, perhaps the most ecstatic of his life, but when it was over, he felt completely empty; he felt like someone alive in a deep-buried coffin. He almost felt like a puppet whose strings were being pulled by some maniacal, grinning thing only half-corporeal.

He could even hear a faint gusting sound, like a drift, an almost inaudible laughing …

At last, his consciousness slid into sleep like a disease insinuating itself, a virus dragging him down into sickness, and once sleep had established itself …

You are Dakuri, and you are the senior prefect for the court of Tiglath III, one of the greatest kings of the Assyrian empire. The king looks on from his high throne of gold and onyx, dressed in multilayered tunics flecked with jewels and a crown of staggered gold stems.

You step forth and bow to your king in the great shining marble room. Soldiers in battle dress flank either side, bearing fiery torches.

The king nods to you and smiles.

As senior prefect, you are also the court's executioner, and executions in ancient Assyria are always preceded by some of the first methods of systemic torture. Children of captured enemy commanders were tied up and lain in piles, to be burned alive while the commanders are forced to watch. The wives of these commanders have their hands, feet, ears, noses, lips, and breasts cut off—slowly—for the entertainment of the court. Then the commanders themselves are skinned and dissected alive, after which diviners, called Exipitrists, toss the intestines on the stone floor and read the king's future in the glistening configuration.

As the king's favorite prefect, you, Dakuri, have perpetrated all of these tortures and many, many more.

No one knows for sure, but some scholars cite the Assyrians as the inventors of the simple head-crusher. A sturdy table with a U-shape cut out on one edge allows an insertion point for the victim's neck. Mounted over this is an iron vise-like contraption with an inverted metal bowl, which fits over the victim's head. The process is quite uncomplicated, actually, and serves as a great spectator event for Assyrian nobility.

And now you, Dakuri, step forth. You come from a long line of court torturers; in fact, your name means "son of the crusher." Now that you've bowed to your king, you approach the table, into which the victim has already been strapped. This one, a comely female, was said to be a Chaldean witch. Her tongue had been cut out at once so she could not intone hexes upon the king, and her hands, too, were amputated to prevent her from making evil signs of imprecation. For a month or two, she's been passed back and forth between the many barracks of the king's body guards; hence, there is little left of her by the time her execution date arrives, and by now, she is surely a little bit pregnant. Two dead Chaldeans are always better than one.

You jam her neck forward and reel down the bowl till it fits over her head. She shrieks and jabbers at you, for those are the only noises she can make now. You grab the wheel and turn it fully once, and this locks her head in tighter. Another turn and the tabletop catches her chin, then another, and her shrieks reduce to whimpers because her teeth are beginning to crumble as her jaw is driven up into her top teeth.

Now your cock is *really* hard, and you know it will get harder still with every further twist of the iron wheel.

The idea is to extend the process as long as possible, in order to keep the prisoner alive the longest and, hence, feel more pain. Another twist and her lips buckle and her neck bends to the left.

Now you turn the wheel in shorter increments. Her body is convulsing now, and a piping, whistling sound escapes her throat. The little bit of water in her bladder empties and collects on the floor. Even this mundane process excites you; you are squeezing the piss out of her, and as you do so, your cock thumps and drools.

Several more minuscule twists of the wheel and you hear that rewarding sound—not a crack, not a snap, but a semi-muffled *thunk,* the sound of the witch's skull experiencing its first buckle. But she's still jittering there, still convulsing, and after a few more cranks, the major sutures of her skull begin to part and the head slowly collapses.

Even when the iron bowl can descend no farther, the woman's body still convulses.

The row of spectators seem in awe, and the king, especially, grins at your regal work. He flips his hand, meaning you can go now, so you bow to him, then hurry out of the chamber. You can't wait to get back to your quarters, to masturbate—

—your name is William Cawler, and you are a sergeant in the 3rd Colorado Cavalry Regiment, and on November 29, 1864, your detachment from Fort Laramie is, in the middle of the night, ordered to attack a non-combatant congregation of Cheyenne Indians; the able-bodied men of this remnant tribe were still out on the hunt, leaving only 600 or so women, children, and elderly.

It's almost a medieval scene when your mounted

platoon arrives. Gunshots pepper the night, fires burn, and some of the fires are people set ablaze. When you and your men dismount, one of your privates exclaims, "Sarge, it ain't but just squaws and kids, babies even. What do we do?" "Kill 'em all," you reply. "That's an order from Colonel Chivington himself. These injuns broke a treaty they signed with the 54th, and bushwhacked a hunnert of our men and a couple 'a wagon trains," but the private looks aghast and tells you, "Sarge, I don't think these are the Indians who did that, these are—" You look the young man right in the eye and say, "Are you disobeyin' a direct order from the colonel?" "I—I ... no. No, sarge." "Good. Then kill every injun you see, squaws, kids, all of 'em, or it's forty lashes."

Orders are orders, you think, *And just be grateful you're here instead of fightin' the johnny rebs,* and with that, you draw your Colt 1851 revolver and blow the head clean off of a Native American woman trying to flee the field. Everywhere you look, Indians are fleeing. None of them have guns. Several old men with tomahawks and old trade axes attack a squad of dismounted troops but are mown down in a hail of thirty-six-caliber bullets. *God damn,* you think, watching troops cut down teepees to let more mounted troops trample them, most of which cover women and children. Muzzle-flash and gunfire do not relent as screams sail across the scene like wind.

Eventually, the chaos begins to fade, and there's not much left alive. You see multiple Native American women dead on the ground, many with child-heavy papooses on their backs—the bullets went through the babies and into the backs of the mothers. Old men lay dead or dying, gargling blood. Your men are not modest—they don't hesitate to drag an attractive squaw off into the shadows to rape. All you do is walk around and stare. What else *can* you do?

Orders are orders, you think.

You help yourself to some jerky you find in a demolished teepee, but then the platoon commander, Lieutenant Norton, grabs your shoulder and excitedly says, "Cawler, come on, there's money ta be made over here," and then you follow him to a patch of scrub beyond the fires, and you see rows and rows of dead Indian children lain out as if for inspection. Several troops are methodically scalping these children with broad-bladed Bowie knives, and it is then that you notice not all of the children are dead, yet their scalps are flensed right off their heads just the same. Some are even babies, their hairless scalps whisked right off as well.

Norton grins at you. "Blade up, Cawler, 'fore it's all gone. Quartermaster knows some fellas who're buyin' chillun's scalps for twenty apiece—"

"Twennie apiece!" you exclaim. "That's crazy!"

"Maybe, but's true. They sell 'em ta collectors in Denver, Carson City, them places." Norton whips out his own Buck knife and starts scalping a little Indian boy, cutting around the ears so they stay connected. "More money if their ears are still on," he says, and then he gets back to cutting.

Well, shit my drawers! you think. *I just knowed this fuckin' Army shit'd pay off some day ...*

Your own Bowie knife glints in distant firelight, and you scalp six kids in a row, lickety-split—three little girls and three little boys—and figuring how to best keep the little ears connected is easier than you thought. Then you think, *What in blazes?* That sixth child, a little girl, is still alive. *Aw, well, ain't nothin' I can do about that,* you realize, and keep cutting—

—while you're feeling up the dead young woman named Lynda in the woods, you think back rather dismally to the one last month. Was her name Joni? Or, no, Karen? You can't remember. You snuck into her basement bedroom, broke off a bedpost, and bashed her in the head with it. Then you tried to fuck her, but …

It wouldn't work. Were you too nervous? Your cock just hung there like a little tadpole, and you imagined, though the front of Joni's head was bashed in, you imagined that she was laughing at you, laughing at your impotence. *Well, fuck that,* you thought, and you decided that if you couldn't fuck her with your cock, you'd fuck her with the bedpost, and you made a great job of *that.* It tore her insides up but good. And you got the last laugh anyway because Joni somehow survived, but as a brain-damaged invalid.

That's what you're thinking about when you're doing the job on this next one, Lynda. You'd seen her at Dante's, drinking with her fussy girlfriends, and you knew at once that you had to have her. You followed her home, waited till everyone was asleep, then you broke in through the side door and bludgeoned her, hard, but not enough to kill her. Bold as brass, you carried the bitch out to the car and drove her up the mountain road to the woods, and that's where you choked her out, stripped her, and played with her body. You fingered her, plied her dead breasts, tongued her dead mouth. You hadn't been this excited since that eight-year-old girl you killed and raped when you were fourteen, the little girl on your paper route.

But you couldn't have this one laughing at you, not Lynda, so you cut off her head with a DeWalt hacksaw and propped the wide-eyed head up so it could watch you fucking her body. This time, you were already rock-hard when you sank it in, and it was a delicious feeling when you came in her. But those orgasms were much *more* delicious when you returned over the next days to fuck her corpse some more.

If fact, there is no better sensation in the world than coming in dead pussy.

Your name is Ted, and you'll leave many more bodies in this same area in the future, and many more heads—

—and when Farthing woke up, he felt like he was drowning in black, putrid quicksand that stank of road-kill in the sun. Revulsion pried his mouth open in a tight gasp, and he thought sure he'd throw up right there in the bed, until the impulse was distracted by the sounds of *someone else* throwing up. He glanced to his right and saw that it was Mal hanging off the edge of the bed, vomiting loudly.

One heave after another. One gust after the next …

Just then, sickened as he was, Farthing felt his groin: he was hard, and there was ample evidence that he'd either masturbated repeatedly or ejaculated in his sleep.

When Mal hauled herself back up, she glared at him with bloodshot eyes and a bright-pink face, puke on her lips. "The bloody hell, Farthing," she croaked.

"You saw it all again?"

"Yes! And it was the worst this time!"

Farthing fell back on the pillows. *Yeah, it was.* "Serves you right. You're the one who said it's an *honor* to see what the Devil has seen," and then he actually laughed.

"Yeah? Well I was wrong. I gotta get out of this shit. I'm in too deep—"

"But you *can't* get out, can you? Not with that belly full of horror, and same for that cunting fourteen-year-old. You're both in for the long haul, just like me. But those assholes out there *need me. Will they really need you and Karen after you drop those babies?"*

Mal's only response was her open stare.

Farthing felt like two people now, two different people mashed together: one, the boring, normal chump who was appalled by all these goings-on, and the opposite, an occult sexual-sociopath, a madman psychically connected to the *princeps tenebrarum.* He gazed at her bare legs, the big belly and tits pushing against the black t-shirt, and the urge returned to fuck her again, put one in her pussy this time and knock on that evil baby's door.

"No," she said, hate in her eyes. "I'm not going through the wringer again, not today, you twisted fuck."

Yeah, I guess I AM a twisted fuck, he consented. He liked Mal, but how could he like her and hate her so much at the same time? Sometimes it felt so good simply to hate everyone.

He got up and peeked out the curtains, astonished that it was late afternoon. "Fuck, we slept all night and then half the day away. It'll be dusk soon. I guess we better get ready." And then he went to the shower.

Farthing just sat in the living room armchair, drinking more beer, staring. Saed, Kirill, Asenieth, and the ever blank-faced Walter were already there, and so was Karen, who rubbed her bulging stomach and smiled each time she glanced at Farthing. In fantasy, Farthing saw himself breaking a two-by-four across her face and then kicking Asenieth between the legs as hard as he could, just

… because.

Two strong men from a caterer's lifted in a sizable mini-bar and set it down in the kitchen, and then they left. It was Kirill—no surprise—who assumed the role of bartender. Farthing winced, looking at his belly. *Jeez, buddy. Your stomach's bigger than Mal and Karen's put together. I guess they don't have Weight Watchers in fuckin' Russia.*

As the sun sank, a loud motor was heard just out front, and then excited talking. Farthing looked out the bow window and saw a Mercedes bus stopped and at least ten more people stepping off and coming into the trailer. The bus drove away when all had disembarked, and in moments, the living room was filled with a yapping polyglot throng. It was like a whack-job reunion: persons of all colors, multiple age groups, an array of international apparel, gleefully snapping at each other in any number of accents. Here was a Kuwaiti oil minister, and there a South Korean CEO. Also, some guy from the Congo in a dashiki and one of those hats that looked like a small waste basket on his head. His skin was black, not dark-brown, but *black*, like anthracite coal. Next, an attractive, smartly dressed woman in her fifties who Farthing could swear he'd seen on the news once, a big wheel in the UN Security Council. Another woman he'd seen on news shows occasionally, who he thought was the prime minister of some smaller country in Europe. Two other well-dressed Americans talked at the drink cart, both middle-aged, one bald as a cue-ball, the other with glasses, no tie, and mussed hair.

Farthing could've laughed as he looked around: a bunch of fussy rich people sipping over-priced wine and chitchatting. *Look at me,* Farthing thought. *I'm sitting in the middle of a satanic cocktail party ...*

The room began to darken as outside did, and the faces of his "guests" darkened too—dark faces showing bright white teeth and glittering eyes. Soon it would be time, Farthing knew, and even as his stomach roiled at the thought, his cock and balls sparked up in abominable expectation.

He'd have to turn on the TV and see more, *more of the worst atrocities ever committed by man. At least the images on the television were without sound, unlike his dreams, but now that he thought about it, perhaps that funeral-parlor soundlessness made it even worse.*

Karen drifted over, grinning as always; her belly and milk-sodden breasts stretched out her maternity dress. "Where's Mal?" she asked.

"Probably hanging herself, which is what you and I should be doing."

"Oh, come on, you love this—the *power* of it all. All these people, some of the richest, most powerful people in the world, and they're all in *awe* of you."

"Then they need their heads examined. So do you."

"For me? I couldn't feel more blessed. Of all the girls in the world, and they pick me," she said. Her eyes seemed alight. "I feel resplendent. My inclusion with the group is sheer serendipity."

Farthing frowned. "For a junior-high teeny-bopper, you sure have a great vocabulary."

She stood up on her tiptoes and grinned even more wolfishly. "This is gonna start soon. Let me blow you first."

"I'd rather put my dick in a dumpster drain."

That put an end to her grin. "You really are a nasty piece-of-shit motherfucker."

"Baby, there's nobody more aware of that than me," Farthing agreed. "Now take your tits and stomach out of my sight."

A little later, Saed looked at his watch and interrupted in a loud voice, "Friends? By the grace of our benefactor ... it's time."

Walter came up behind Farthing, grabbed his shoulder, and nudged him toward the back room. The others finished their drinks and followed in a sudden silence that was somehow echoic and ghastly.

Farthing knew his place by now; he sat down in the metal chair before the old television. Everyone else stood behind him—the room was packed. Saed stood just before the television, facing the congregation like a reverend in a church. "On this darkest and holiest of nights, my brothers and sisters, we gather to behold yet again this great miracle and the proof of our living lord."

Silence. Then:

The congregation, in unison, asked, "Shall we have it?"

Saed responded resonantly: "Thou wilt."

"Shall we amass wealth and be envied?"

"Thou wilt."

"Shall we die peaceably in our beds, slaked of loins and with bellies full of ambrosia? And shall we descend to live in paradise forever?"

"Thou shalt," Saed replied. "And if a man or woman desireth a long life and wouldst kill thine enemies without forethought, and if they would drinketh the blood of the foul and dare to behold visions most abominable, thou must make sacrifice and salute the Regia Aeris with a whole heart, and bowest down in blessedness."

"So let it be so, in joyous darkness."

"O friend and ruler of night, thou who

rejoicest in the baying of dogs and spilt blood, who wanderest in the midst of shades among the tombs, who longst for blood and bringest terror to mortals, look favorably on our reverence."

"So let it be so, in joyous darkness."

"Father of the Earth, as you see the Earth through us, let us see it ourselves, through you."

The congregation finished by chanting, "*Pater Terrae, Per Me Vide Terrum.*"

Farthing dismissed the orison as a hokey joke, but then why did he feel suddenly euphoric?

A shadow came up from behind, then skirted around to stand before him. It was Mal, buck naked, stomach stretched forth so tight and shiny that Farthing could almost see his semi-reflection in it.

She was holding a cup, not a paper cup but an ornate cup of black stone.

"Shit, Mal …"

"Just drink it," she said. "Someday you'll be rewarded like you could never imagine, and so will I."

"You believe that shit?" Farthing said, already half-hard by looking at her body. "From the Prince of *Lies?*"

"Drink it. Or Walter will make you."

Farthing supposed she was right; he saw Walter

looking at him with his one eye, a hand over the scabbarded knife under his jacket.

Mal put the cup to his lips and tipped it. Farthing drank gustily. The hot metallic liquid shot down his throat and filled his stomach, where it seemed to buzz and pulsate. He wanted to throw it all back up onto her bulging stomach, and vomit some more upa in Saed's face, and in Kirill's and Asenieth's, and right on the head of that evil little cunt Karen … but only an instant later, that *other* part of himself began to resurface, and with it so did his lust, his greed, and his hatred. Now his cock was so hard it hurt. The room's single light seemed to dim, and the silent static bloomed on the old television, and he had the feeling now that his spirit, if he had one, was being sucked into it—

—and here you are now, with a delirious grin, naked and your erection sticking out like a prong, fucking, fucking, fucking, any available hole amongst the carpet of squirming humans at the Chapel of Our Lady of Endor, the marble halls of the Order of the Black Sun, the naves of Wycombe, and the suburban carpets of NXIVM. That's what it's all about: fucking, sex, having orgasms. Men, women, it doesn't matter. You serve Iblis by offending God, and you offend God by fucking everything that moves. Cum flying. Ejaculation after ejaculation. Waste the precious seed and exploit others for your own pleasure because *that* is what the world is. The women below you have been fucked raw yet still they grin, still they gasp for more, and you will bury your cock into each and every one of their bloody pussies, fill them up with cum, and move on to the next, all in the name of—

—and then you are dragged off, as if by a handful of hair, as if through a black tarn, and next thing you know, you're in one of the outbuildings just beyond the camp. Now your name is Norio Nakaya, and you are a captain in the Imperial Japanese Army and the highest ranking man on the island. With your sharpened bayonet, you are cutting the calf and quadricep muscles off of a former soldier, either from India or Singapore, allied to the despicable British. There's not much meat left on these prisoners, no, not in 1944, and not after years of slave labor building landing strips on Papau. You started with several thousand, but now you're down to several hundred—starvation is the chief cause of death. Rations, once abundant and actively resupplied, are down to nearly nothing. In the past, each prisoner was allotted a pound of rice flour every day, as well as several ounces of dog meat or fish, and some vegetables when they were procurable (after all, how well could prisoners work if malnourished?). But now that the tides have turned, you have had to cut prisoner rations down to three ounces of flour, and that was all, and even that won't last much longer.

You and your squad of guards have no choice but to eat the meat of prisoners who are no longer strong enough to work. Each day you pick a few who look least likely to live much longer. You drag them to the outbuilding and cut the meat off their bones while they're still alive. They scream loud and hard, and you want that, you *want* the prisoners in the camp to hear the screams, and when you begin cooking the meat (which has an aroma like roast pork), you *want* that smell to drift across the camp so the starving prisoners know what's happening. You also cut out the hearts and livers and cook those as well. The liver is especially important, and it tastes better than anything else. Throughout history, the patricial Japanese believed that the liver was the organ that contained courage and loyalty, and the heart contained the soul, and that the greatest demonstration of victory is eating the flesh of your enemies.

Well, you don't know about all that, but you

do know that if you don't consume enough meat every day, then you will not be able to fulfill your obligation to the Emperor. So you eat, and you eat with a smile of gratitude on your face. Every now and then, the gods reward you for your diligence: downed American fliers wash up on the island. They're strapping and healthy, and you put them to work … but always take one aside so you can cut off all that delectable muscle meat and fill your bellies—

—now you're eating more human flesh, but your name isn't Norio Nakaya, it's Jeffrey Dahmer, and you're really off your rocker. Though you tried to eat one victim's dick once (it wasn't very good), your favorite part is the bicep. To you, the bicep is what makes the man most attractive; it's the symbol of his masculine strength, and that's what you want *in you*, so that he is not forgotten, so that he is not relegated to oblivion. Just as you've read in books, it tastes pretty much like the meat of a pork chop.

All your men are beautiful, and they try to escape when they can, and that's the part that hurts you. Why don't they want to stay? For your whole life, everyone has left you. In the future, when you're caught, people will think that you *like* killing them, but that's actually the part you hate. Several times you drilled holes in their skulls and put stuff in the holes—acid, a few drops of boiling water, carpet nails—because you thought that would sort of lobotomize them and take away their desire to abandon you.

Little do you know, you are actually engaging in an ancient practice called trepanation. People in olden times would have holes cut into their heads to relieve headaches because they thought the headaches were caused by evil spirits, and those evil spirits would leave through the hole. Well, in that case, maybe you should just drill a hole in *your own* head …

You like to jerk off with their severed hands or cum on their dead body parts. You don't precisely remember the first time you sucked a dead man's cock nor fucked a dead man's ass, but you do remember the power of it, and the comfort: knowing that they would not abandon you—

—favorite thing to do in the field is ordering your men to smash the knees and ankles of your captives—mostly women, children, and old men—to drag them screaming into the church, and to chain the doors shut. Then your underlings set the church on fire, and you and your men sit down on the ground to watch. It's like a picnic.

You are a child-rapist named Oskar Dirlewanger, and you have been released from prison—ironically, Welzheim concentration camp—thanks to the influence of your old NSDAP friend, General Berger. It is Berger's idea to form special penal combat units to unloose in Poland and Belarus, and to slaughter civilians who might join in local resistance activities. Berger chooses *you* to command this first brigade that will become famously known as the Dirlewanger Brigade, and you are promoted to the esteemed rank of SS-Oberführer.

Quite an achievement for a child-rapist.

Uniquely, your brigade is composed of hardened criminals released from incarceration on the condition that they kill for the Fatherland. They are mostly poachers, psychotics, murderers, and, yes, more child-molesters. The idea is to exterminate civilians in these sub-human outlands, especially children before the degenerates can mature and reproduce to make more enemies of the Reich. So there you have it. You go from scum of the earth to decorated SS commander in charge of helping fulfill Der Führer's order for proper living space for true Germans.

And you now have *carte blanche* to fuck and kill

every little girl in eastern Europe.

Burning civilians alive inside churches is one pastime activity while in the field, but when you're on a weekend pass, your favorite thing to do is kidnap a young girl, strip her, and rape her repeatedly; when you can't come anymore, you inject her with half a milligram of strychnine and just sit back and watch, fondling your exhausted genitals as the girl first begins to vomit uncontrollably, voids her bowels, and then goes into catastrophic seizures. Her back and legs arch to an impossible degree, her eyes bleed, her hands and feet cramp into fists, and her jaw clamps shut so hard her teeth break. Then she begins to spasm into a repertoire of cringing poses. Doctors have told you it's like a full-body charley-horse that can't be relieved, and you delight in the idea of inflicting that much pain upon a child. Best are the facial muscle cramps that draw the face into an insane, grinning rictus. Eventually, most victims die because the throat muscles close off the airway, and those that don't, you hang with piano wire.

Little do you know that in August, 1944, while engaged in "counter-insurgency" operations near Warsaw, your unit will seize a daycare facility full of 500 children under the age of six. You order them all killed but only with blunt objects and rifle butts because you need to conserve ammunition, and you do similar things in Slovakia and Hungary. For your gallant service, you are awarded the Knight's Cross of the Iron Cross, and the SS-Sturmbrigade Dirlewanger will be credited with murdering at least 40,000 civilians—

—name is Willy, but they call you "Rat" on the cell block because you have a shitty-looking little ponytail type thing hanging off the back of your head that looks like a rat-tail, and you're balding, and your eyes are disturbingly close together due to remnant inbreeding in your hereditary past.

Though you'd committed many crimes before the age of twenty-five (theft, burglary, assault with intent to kill, and, especially, child molestation), you somehow managed *never* to get caught. Even more miraculously, at about that age, you are hired as a night-shift janitor at a maternity hospital. Of course, they background-check you, but you pass with flying colors!

There are multiple baby wards in the hospital, each with a nursing station where there is always someone, usually a CNA, making rounds of the ward 24/7 and checking any outbursts of crying, even in the middle of the night. But in truth, her main task is to change diapers, and *your* main job is to wheel the sack down to the laundry when it's full. You suppose it's that sweet aroma of baby feces that does it. It really gets into your head and gets your cock leaking. It makes you *hard,* and you always have to jerk off after taking a sack down, and you don't think about any of those cutie-pie CNAs, you think about the babies.

Sometimes you daydream and actually remember things from a long time ago. Can people remember things that happened back when they were three and four years old? Well, you're sure *you* can, and you remember how your stepmother hated to hear her babies cry—she had two of them, one six months, one a year and a half. But you were a *good* little boy and *never* cried; she'd tell you so many times.

At any rate, you remember sitting in your highchair and watching her grasp each crying baby's head in her hands, and then she'd shake shake shake that head so vigorously that the head and her hands blurred, and she did it to each baby's head for several minutes, and suddenly their heads would just loll on their necks and they'd stare upward open-mouthed, and she'd use an eyedropper to give them whiskey too, and between that and the head-shaking, they'd *never* cry again. And you had a pretty good idea why *you* never cried as a baby either.

So when you get older, you hear about it and read about it: Shaken Baby Syndrome. It warps their soft skulls and bruises their brains and causes all kind of mental problems and learning disabilities when they're older. In other words, it fucks those babies *all up* for the rest of their lives.

And you *like* that idea. Because you know *you* got all fucked up too.

One of your neighbors is a drug-dealer named Kip, and when you say you want to buy stuff to make people fall asleep, he sells you this stuff called doxepin. "Just put a quarter of one of these caps in their drink, and they'll be out for an hour or more," Kip promises.

This is something you've been thinking about for a long time …

Katie always works mid-to-eights on D Ward. She's pretty and has big tits, and you can see her nipples through her white top a little bit, but you don't really care. "Willy?" she says as she has many times, "Could you get me a coffee from the automat? And get something for you too." "Sure, Miss Katie," you say. "Cream and sugar, right?" "Yeah, thanks." You take the offered money and leave, and get to the automat quickly without looking conspicuous. You get her coffee, drop in a quarter of the powder from the pill, and put in the sugar and cream. You taste it with your finger and detect nothing. You buy yourself a bag of chips.

When you deliver her coffee, she lowers her voice as she talks on her cellphone. Maybe she's talking about you—you know you're a little funny looking—but you could care less. Probably a boyfriend she's talking to, someone she's fucking. Maybe she'll get pregnant, have the baby, then you can *fuck* that baby up too. But you let the fantasy go. You've got work to do!

You disappear and mop the main hall, then you look back at the nurse's station and there's Katie, face down on the desk. You're inside the ward in a heartbeat, shaking babies' heads as fast and as hard as you can. One after another after another. Shake-shake-shake-shake-shake-shake, and on and on and on, until you've fucked up all twenty babies on the ward. They'll be mentally retarded. They won't be able to talk right or learn right. You beam proudly at yourself when you think of what you've just done, and now you're gonna do it all the time. You're gonna fuck up as many babies as you can, just like the world fucked *you* up.

"Miss Katie?" you say, tapping her shoulder an hour later. "Wake up now."

"Whuh … Huh?" she murmurs and brings her

head off the desk.

"You fell asleep. But don't worry, no one saw."

"Aw, shit." She looks up at you, pleadingly. "Please don't tell anyone, Willy. I'd get fired."

"Of course I'd never tell no one," you assure her. "See ya later." Then you push your mop cart away to the next ward.

You'll do the same thing various times on various wards for the next year: fucking up a couple *hundred babies.*

But, alas, no party lasts forever, does it? Eventually, you get caught when one of the CNAs wakes up too early, screams so loud everyone on the floor hears, and when the security guys barge in, what they see in the ward glass is: you, with a baby's head in your hands, grinning maniacally, shaking shaking shaking shaking—

—feels like Farthing is throwing up diarrhea, his eyes bugging, and he has the sense of falling as if he'd been holding on to a rope off a great precipice and then that rope was *cut—*

Farthing is falling, traversing in the air, hair flying. Are those gunshots he hears? Are those screams? His memory is pitch-black and percolating, bubbling like hot tar, but then images begin to surface with each popping bubble:

Dirlewanger, Dahmer, the Indian massacre and scalping party, and on and on, everything Farthing was forced to watch on that infernal television and was forced to show others. He knows full well that a world with things like that in it is no world for him. But finally, there is some solace. He can end it all by blowing his head off with that big pistol hidden under the patio tile, can't he?

The last black bubble of tar pops, and he sees not the defective madman named Rat shaking all those babies by the head but—

Aw, fuck this. I'm punching out …

—himself, Farthing, grinning insanely and shake-shake-shaking those babies by their heads and damaging them, fucking them up, demonstrating Lucifer's perfect distillation of evil.

And then, tears in his eyes, he stops falling, and he is lying on his back in a narrow bed, staring up. He tastes puke in his mouth and his stomach is convulsing and his ears are ringing and—

EPILOGUE

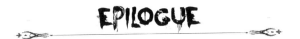

"There he is, the man of the hour," came a snide male voice in a British accent.

Farthing didn't know where he was, but he wouldn't have to wonder long before all would be made clear to him.

He could hear his eyes click when he blinked, and his ears were distantly ringing. When he sat up, collected himself, and looked around, he realized he was sitting up on a metal-framed cot-like bed in a room made of shiny cinderblocks. Next to him was a stainless-steel toilet and sink, and the front wall of this cubicle was made of iron bars.

The snide Brit, of course, proved to be a uniformed detention officer.

When Farthing's train of thought began to

unclog, he snapped, "What am I doing here?"

"Ah, gonna play that card, eh?" The guard smiled, tapping his foot. "Pretend to be crazy? The devil made me do it? I heard voices? Well, maybe that works over the pond where you're from, but it don't take over here. You're in bev-seg right now, but we'll do everything we can to get'cha into the mainstream prison population. Fellas like you get quite the pranging in general pop. Won't take long before your asrehole's big enough to park a double-decker in."

Farthing only half heard him through the clamor of his own confusion. "I don't get it. What did I do? I remember ... being in the trailer ..."

"Yeah, you were in the trailer, all right, mate. Killed everyone in it with a big old Webley, the bobbies say. Then you dumped petrol from the garden shed all over the bodies and inside but"— the guard laughed out loud—"you couldn't find a bloomin' lighter! Can you imagine that?"

Farthing sat upright on the edge of the cot, his mind ticking. *Did I really? Did I kill them all?* "Please. Tell me exactly what I did."

"You pullin' me leg?" said the guard. "Guess not, but, sure, I'll tell ya. First, you shot two billionaires—that's right, *billionaires*. Some guy from one 'a them oil countries, Kuwait or Emerites or some shit, and one 'a them Russian *oolagarks,* docked his hundred-million-pound yacht at the fuckin' Burnstow marina. Ya shot one in the crotch, and the big bullet went right through and through the other one too—they both bled out on the floor. Then there was some ex-con with an eye-patch; you shot him in his *good* eye, you did, put his brains all over the walls."

Farthing didn't remember. Saed, Kirill, and Walter. He'd fantasized about killing them, hadn't he? But why couldn't he remember?

"Wait a minute!" he rushed. "The Turkish woman, Asenieth? Did I shoot her too?"

"The defense minister, kind of a looker?" Another laugh from the guard. "You sure did. Ya bent her over the couch and shot her right in the pussy. The bobbies say the bullet came out her mouth. That's a piece 'a work, that is."

Farthing's shoulders slumped. *Wow. I guess it's all true.* If there was one thing Farthing could genuinely see himself doing, it would be shooting that vulture Asenieth right between the legs.

Fuck, I'm in deep trouble.

"So, tell me something, mate?" asked the guard. "It's everybody's guess. What's a couple 'a billionaires and a Turkish defense minister doing with the likes of you in a bloody retirement trailer?"

"You won't believe me," Farthing answered. "Want me to tell you anyway?"

The guard grinned. "Sure."

"They came to watch the television."

"Did they now?"

"Not the big television in the living room, the old one in the back room. See, only I can turn it on."

"Um-hmm. I see."

"And those people I killed, there were a bunch more there too, but they must've left after the show was over—I can only keep the TV on for as long as the blood lasts."

"Of course! That don't sound daft at all!"

"They're all satanists, some kind of a global network, I think."

The guard held out his palms. "And there ya have it! Mystery solved. It was a *satanic network* what made you kill them people—"

Another jolt of alarm. "Wait a minute! Did I destroy the television? Please tell me I destroyed the television!"

"Oh, right. The bobbies who brought you in, they *did say something about a telly in the back room. Oldest telly they ever seen, they said—*"

"Did I destroy it!?"

The guard amusedly shook his head. "Ya tried to,

mate. Ya dumped petrol all over it and everything else, but like I just told you, you couldn't find a lighter. That's what I call paralyzed from the neck up."

Fuuuuuuck ...

"So what's the big deal about the telly?"

Farthing couldn't resist smiling at him. "It only shows the worst atrocities in the history of mankind. How's that for an answer?"

"Wow, mate. You think that up all by yourself? Good luck with that one in court."

Then, something slammed in Farthing's head. "Oh my God ... Mal, and Karen—I didn't kill *them,* did I? There's no way I would've—"

"Them two birds who was preggo?" The guard nodded slowly, grinning. "Killed 'em both, shot 'em right in the stomach. I mean, tell me somethin', mate. What kind 'a *man* shoots pregnant women in the stomach?"

Farthing instantly buried his face in his hands. *No, no, I couldn't have ...*

"And one of 'em was fourteen, they told me—a fuckin' *child.* Yes, sir, you get my vote for Man of the Year."

So I killed Mal and Karen AND the two babies ...

Suddenly it occurred to him why he would do such a thing. To end Eldred's line, to make it so no one would ever see the shit on that television again. *With both babies dead, the line ends with me. And, come to think of it, I'm GLAD I had the balls to kill those other evil fuckers.*

"But ya did get a speck of luck from somewhere," the guard went on. "You'll only get one infanticide conviction. See, the fourteen-year-old's baby lived, bullet never even hit it. Went under its chin, they said. It miscarried right as the first-responders was comin' in, and they saved it. God be praised, eh?"

Farthing stared into cinderblocks. He seriously doubted that God had anything to do with it.

"And ya lucked out even more," continued the guard. "The UK ain't all savage-like, not like the US. We abolished the death penalty way back in the sixties. Now, you ask me, we ought to bring it back for blokes like you—death by woodchipper, I say. And I'd be the first to volunteer pushin' the button." The guard sighed. "Ah, but I guess it's better for you to just do life. Worst thing to be in stir, mate, is a baby-killer. Those fellas? They'll fuck your arsehole inside out, they will, and I hope you like the taste 'a cum 'cos your life's about to become an all-you-can-swallow buffet."

Terrific, Farthing thought. And I guess that's that.

The guard left, chuckling.

At least Farthing didn't feel bad about killing

Saed and his scumbag friends. It had to have been the television that pushed him over the edge. The last fiber of anything decent left in him took charge and did the job … But it was too bad about Mal and Karen. He'd actually kind of liked Mal.

Might as well make the best of it, he thought in the tinted darkness. And at least I'll never have to watch that fuckin' television again. Won't have to drink any more dirty blood and perform for satanic psychos like a chimp at the circus.

So it was true: no more atrocities on that television—the fuckin' *telly.*

But there was no getting away from it, not really, and this he would find out later that night, when he fell asleep and saw it all over and over again in his dreams, everything and more, every horror the human mind had ever dreamed up and ever would, every night for the rest of his life.

Not all that much later, and not all that far off, quite a few very expensive automobiles pulled up in front of an opulent suburban house and stopped. From every car, an assemblage of remarkably well-dressed persons disembarked and proceeded for the front door.

Was a baby heard crying inside?

Perhaps.

Not long afterwards, a delivery truck backed up into the driveway. The rear door slid open, and then a bevy of sturdy young moving men carefully lifted something out of the back of the truck: a very, very old television set.

AUTHOR'S NOTE

More than likely, some of you (hopefully a great many) are familiar with English academic and ghost-story writer M.R. James. The work of Dr. James means a great deal to me, such that I read passages of his nearly every night, for over the last twenty-five years. Eccentric, I know. I rank James second only to Lovecraft as history's most important scribe of horror (In fact, I reread Lovecraft almost constantly as well). But I've reread James more than any other author, and I think it's because I'm enthralled by the man's "prose-intellect," if you will, and the obvious manner with which he celebrates the full wonders of the English language in the composition of his stories. Like Lovecraft, James took the use of words very seriously and took great pains to make sure that the "right ones" found their way onto the page. Beyond this, I'm at a loss to put you in possession of my indefatigable obsession with M.R. James.

It makes sense that, having reread SO MUCH James in my life, aspects of the great man's style might infect my own, and this, I'm afraid, is quite the case. I can't help it; it's almost as if the mechanics of James's style has become imbued into my creative DNA, and if you read this book—and hopefully finish it—those of you who are James afficionados will notice how liberally I have borrowed aspects of James's most characteristic turns of phrase, sentence structures, and other creative flourishes. Detractors will call this a rip-off, but I assure you that it's not and that I'm trying to deceive no one. And though I gravely suspect that Dr. James would NOT approve of the plot and details of this book, I believe he would be positive and amused by this demonstration of my love for the way he wrote. So I guess that's what this is, my tribute, my love letter, to Montague Rhodes James.

E.L.

WHO IS EDWARD LEE?

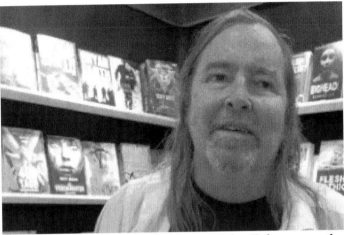

Edward Lee, with collaborator John Pelan, won the first two official Gross Out contests in 1996 and 1997, for passages from their co-written novella GOON. Lee is the author of over 50 horror, fantasy, and sci-fi novels, and dozens of short stories. He has also had comic scripts published by DC Comics, Verotik Inc., and Cemetery Dance. Many of his novels have been reprinted in Germany, Poland, Japan, Italy, Romania, Greece, the Ukraine, Russia, Spain, and other countries. He is a Bram Stoker Award Nominee; his Lovecraftian novel INNSWICH HORROR won the 2010 Vincent Price Award for Best Foreign Book (Austria), his novel WHITE TRASH GOTHIC won the 2018 Splatterpunk Award for Best Extreme Horror Novel, and his collaborative novella HEADER 3 (with Ryan Harding) won for Best Extreme Novella. In 2020, Lee won the J.F. Gonzales Lifetime Achievement Award. In 2009, the movie version of his novella HEADER was released by Synapse Films; several of his novels are currently under option. Lee is a U.S. Army veteran and lives in Seminole, Florida.

More Books from

Madness Heart Press

Czech Extreme by Edward Lee
isbn: 978-1-955745-06-2

The Bighead by Edward Lee
isbn: 978-1-955745-22-2

Extinction Peak by Lucas Mangum
isbn: 979-8-689548-65-4

You Will Be Consumed by Nikolas Robinson
isbn: 978-1-7348937-7-9

Curse of the Ratman by Jay Wilburn
isbn: 978-1-955745-19-2

Trench Mouth by Christine Morgan
isbn: 978-1-7348937-9-3

Warlock Infernal by Christine Morgan
isbn: 978-1-955745-24-6

Addicted to the Dead by Shane McKenzie
isbn: 978-1-955745-15-4

Muerte con Carne by Shane McKenzie
isbn: 978-1-955745-33-8